EAT SO WHAT!
THE SCIENCE OF WATER-SOLUBLE VITAMINS

EVERYTHING YOU NEED TO KNOW ABOUT VITAMINS B AND C

LA FONCEUR

Copyright © 2024 La Fonceur

All rights reserved.

No part of this publication may be reproduced, stored in a retrieval system or transmitted in any form or by any means, electronic, mechanical, photocopying, recording or otherwise, without prior permission of author.

This book has been published with all efforts taken to make the material error-free. The information on this book is not intended or implied to be a substitute for diagnosis, prognosis, treatment, prescription, and/or dietary advice from a licensed health professional. Author and publisher don't assume and hereby disclaim any liability to any party for any loss, damage, or disruption caused by errors or omissions, whether such errors or omissions result from negligence, accident, or any other cause.

While every effort has been made to avoid any mistake or omission, this publication is being sold on the condition and understanding that neither the author nor the publishers or printers would be liable in any manner to any person by reason of any mistake or omission in this publication or for any action taken or omitted to be taken or advice rendered or accepted on the basis of this work. Some contents that are available in electronic books may not be available in print, or vice versa.

CONTENTS

Preface	iv
UNIT 1: BASICS OF WATER-SOLUBLE VITAMINS	**1**
Chapter 1: Basics of Water-Soluble Vitamins	2
Chapter 2: Not True Vitamins But Still Vitamins!	10
UNIT 2: B VITAMINS	**15**
Chapter 1: Vitamin B1	**16**
1. Everything You Need to Know About Vitamin B1	17
2. Importance of Vitamin B1	27
3. 10 Richest Vegetarian Sources of Vitamin B1	35
Chapter 2: Vitamin B2	**41**
1. Everything You Need to Know About Vitamin B2	42
2. Importance of Vitamin B2	54
3. 10 Richest Vegetarian Sources of Vitamin B2	64
Chapter 3: Vitamin B3	**71**
1. Everything You Need to Know About Vitamin B3	72
2. Importance of Vitamin B3	80
3. 10 Richest Vegetarian Sources of Vitamin B3	90
Chapter 4: Vitamin B5	**98**
1. Everything You Need to Know About Vitamin B5	99
2. Importance of Vitamin B5	107
3. 10 Richest Vegetarian Sources of Vitamin B5	116
Chapter 5: Vitamin B6	**123**
1. Everything You Need to Know About Vitamin B6	124
2. Importance of Vitamin B6	133
3. 10 Richest Vegetarian Sources of Vitamin B6	143

Chapter 6: Vitamin B7 — 150
1. Everything You Need to Know About Vitamin B7 — 151
2. Importance of Vitamin B7 — 159
3. 10 Richest Vegetarian Sources of Vitamin B7 — 165

Chapter 7: Vitamin B9 — 172
1. Everything You Need to Know About Vitamin B9 — 173
2. Importance of Vitamin B9 — 184
3. 10 Richest Vegetarian Sources of Vitamin B9 — 192

Chapter 8: Vitamin B12 — 199
1. Everything You Need to Know About Vitamin B12 — 200
2. Importance of Vitamin B12 — 214
3. 10 Richest Vegetarian Sources of Vitamin B12 — 222

Unit 3: Vitamin C — 228
1. Everything You Need to Know About Vitamin C — 229
2. Importance of Vitamin C — 237
3. 10 Richest Vegetarian Sources of Vitamin C — 247

UNIT 4: VITAMIN COMBINATIONS – DOS AND DON'TS — 256
Vitamin Combinations for Synergistic Health Benefits — 257

Potentially Dangerous Vitamin Combinations You Should Avoid — 262

UNIT 5: DIET PLAN — 264

UNIT 6: RECIPES — 271
Soybean Salad — 272
Vegetable Paneer Tikka — 274
Masala Uttapam — 276
Peanut Chutney — 278
Mixed Dal — 280
Herbed Brown Rice — 282

Nutty Cold Coffee	283
Read Previous Books of The Eat So What! Series	*284*
References	*285*
About The Author	*300*
Read More from La Fonceur	*301*
Connect with La Fonceur	*302*

PREFACE

You may come across countless articles promoting the benefits of vitamins, and they often end with recommendations for specific supplements. Vitamins are often misused by dietary supplement manufacturers and health promoters.

B vitamins are not just for providing energy, nor is vitamin C just for boosting immunity. Water-soluble vitamins play a huge role in your body and are essential for your internal integrity. Once you get to know water-soluble vitamins in-depth, you will be surprised to know how much control you can have over your body with these vitamins.

Nowadays, you can find dietary supplements for almost everything. They are meant to fulfill temporary needs; you cannot rely solely on them. This is because many nutrients can give you several health benefits when you get them through natural food, but when you take supplements of these nutrients, they are unable to provide you the same result. Nature provides you with all the necessary vitamins and won't let you suffer from any vitamin deficiency, provided you are well aware of your vitamin sources. Unless your health care provider prescribes a dietary supplement for a medical condition or deficiency, it is best to rely on natural foods to meet your nutrient needs. Although supplements may be beneficial, they are not regulated by the FDA, and overdose is common and dangerous.

Chronic diseases like diabetes, hypertension, cognitive disorders, arthritis, and cancer are the major health issues in today's world. Our lifestyle and food choices contribute a lot to the development of these chronic diseases. Some poor lifestyle choices we make voluntarily, some we are forced to make due to life priorities at different stages of life, but the least discussed reason is that we are not fully aware of our food, and this involuntarily leads to inadequate nutrition, which contributes a lot to the onset of various diseases, which you could have controlled if you had known better.

When you are deeply aware of the "when," "what," and "how much" of vitamins, you can plan your diet that protect you from various known and unknown diseases. Consuming vitamins from natural sources can provide various health benefits that may surprise you. These vitamins are known to affect your health in various ways, some of which have yet to be fully discovered. This is why relying on vitamin supplements may not provide the same results that can be easily achieved through natural sources. If you are not focusing on getting your essential vitamins from food, you are missing out on many potential health benefits.

As I always emphasize, prevention is better than cure, **Eat So What! The Science of Water-Soluble Vitamins** book focuses on increasing your internal body endurance, boosting your body's defense system, and protecting the integrity of your genetic material, which helps keep chronic diseases at bay.

In this book, you'll learn in-depth about each water-soluble vitamin's critical role in maintaining good health and the latest scientific findings that may influence your vitamin decisions. Although there are only 13 officially established essential vitamins, many unofficial or previously named but now removed vitamins play major roles in your health. Just because they are not established doesn't mean they aren't necessary. We will discuss them one by one, what they are, their role, and through which foods you can increase your unestablished vitamin intake.

We will also look at the benefits of combining specific vitamins for optimal health benefits, as well as the potential consequences of taking certain vitamins with particular foods or medications. This book guides you about both beneficial and harmful combinations of vitamins.

Most importantly, you will get to know which of the richest vegetarian sources can fulfill your Vitamin B and C requirements. By consuming these foods, you can avoid vitamin deficiencies and improve your overall health, reducing your chances of infections and chronic diseases such as cancer, diabetes, high blood pressure, and cognitive disorders. Finally, we will cook some delicious and easy vegetarian recipes that help you maximize the health benefits of vitamins B and C.

Let's start our journey of water-soluble vitamins!

UNIT 1
BASICS OF WATER-SOLUBLE VITAMINS

Chapter 1
BASICS OF WATER-SOLUBLE VITAMINS

Vitamins are organic compounds that your body needs in small quantities to perform various physiological functions. They can be essential or non-essential. Essential nutrients are those your body cannot produce but are crucial for normal body function, so they must be obtained through food.

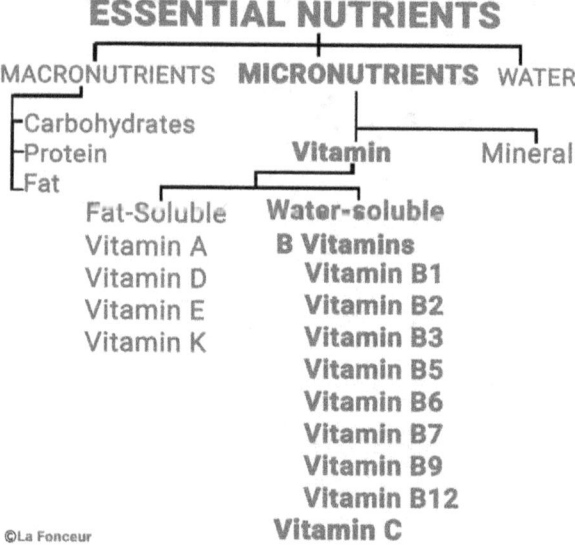

Vitamins are classified as micronutrients because they are required in small quantities. However, this does not make them any less important than macronutrients, such as carbohydrates, proteins, and fats, which are the main energy sources.

CLASSIFICATION OF ESSENTIAL VITAMINS

There are a total of thirteen essential vitamins that are categorised as water-soluble vitamins and fat-soluble vitamins.

Water-Soluble Vitamins

Water-soluble vitamins are vitamin B1, B2, B3, B5, B6, B7, B9, B12 and Vitamin C. These vitamins are called water-soluble as they dissolve in water. There are nine of them, including Vitamin B1 to B12 and Vitamin C. Since they dissolve in water, they are easily absorbed, and any excess amount is excreted in urine quickly without being stored in your body. This is why it is important to consume water-soluble vitamins regularly to maintain adequate levels.

Fat-Soluble Vitamins

Fat-soluble vitamins are vitamins A, D, E, and vitamin K. Fat-soluble vitamins are not soluble in water but dissolve in fats. There are five vitamins that are classified as fat-soluble vitamins - vitamins A, D, E, and K, and the body absorbs these in a similar way to dietary fats. Fat-soluble vitamins A, D, E, and K are stored in the body and can be used whenever your body requires them. This means a continuous supply of fat-soluble vitamins is unnecessary, as they are not excreted from the body as quickly as water-soluble vitamins. However, consuming adequate amounts is important to reach the daily recommended intake.

Fat-soluble vitamins were already discussed in detail in the previous book of this series, "Eat So What! The Science of Fat-Soluble Vitamins." In this book, we will discuss water-soluble vitamins in detail. But first, let us have brief information about water-soluble vitamins, and then we will understand them in detail in the following chapters.

Why do I need water-soluble vitamins?

Your body needs water-soluble vitamins to convert carbohydrates, proteins, and fats into cells' energy currency, i.e., adenosine triphosphate (ATP). These molecules are responsible for supplying energy for various processes in your body. Water-soluble vitamins are also needed to manufacture hemoglobin, boost immune function, and form normal healthy red blood cells (RBCs) that carry oxygen to all the tissues and organs in your body. They are also essential for keeping homocysteine levels within the normal range.

What happens if I am deficient in water-soluble vitamins?

Water-soluble vitamins are vital for the normal functioning of your body. A deficiency in water-soluble vitamins disrupts the internal integrity of the body, which can lead to anemia, eye disorders, cardiovascular diseases, and neurological disorders.

Which water-soluble vitamin deficiency is most common?

Vitamin B12 deficiency is the most common of the water-soluble vitamins. It is usually low in older people and vegans, babies of vegan mothers, vegetarians, or anyone who consumes little or no milk and other animal products. Vitamin B12 is primarily present in animal products, including milk, and its absorption in your body decreases as you age due to reduced gastric acid production.

Types of Water-Soluble Vitamin Deficiencies

There are two types of vitamin deficiencies:

Primary deficiencies are caused by poor diet.

Secondary deficiencies are caused by poor vitamin absorption due to malabsorption, the use of certain medications, and certain medical conditions.

Do water-soluble vitamins have antioxidant properties?

Oxidation is a normal process in your body that provides energy for many cellular functions. It also produces free radicals as a by-product. In small amounts, free radicals are not harmful. Your body has its own antioxidant defense system that kills free radicals. However, when excessive free radicals are produced that exceed your body's natural antioxidants, they start pairing with electrons in fat tissue, proteins, and DNA, and this can damage cells and tissues, increasing the risk of developing chronic diseases like rheumatoid arthritis (RA), cancer, cataracts, diabetes, and neurodegenerative diseases.

Learn about oxidative stress, antioxidants, and inflammation in detail in "Eat So What! The Science of Fat-Soluble Vitamins."

Many of the B vitamins help maintain your body's antioxidant defense system and indirectly promote antioxidant activities. However, only vitamin C is labeled as an antioxidant because it acts as a powerful antioxidant both directly and indirectly. It directly kills free radicals as well as regenerates other antioxidants to provide enhanced action against free radicals and prevent oxidative stress. Vitamin C significantly strengthens your immune system and enhances your body's natural defense. Since your body cannot produce vitamin C, you must obtain it through the diet.

FORTIFIED FOODS

Although food fortification is discussed in detail in "Eat So What! The Science of Fat-Soluble Vitamins," here I am briefly reminding you about fortified foods.

(Skip this section if you have already read "Eat So What! The Science of Fat-Soluble Vitamins.")

What is Food Fortification?

Food fortification and food enrichment sound similar, but the two are different. Both involve adding essential nutrients such as vitamins and minerals to food and share the common goal of preventing nutritional deficiencies and promoting public health. However, food enrichment adds back essential nutrients lost during processing, whereas fortification adds additional essential nutrients that may not be present or may only be present in small amounts before processing.

Two types of food fortification are mandatory fortification, which is done by the government, where food manufacturers are legally obligated to add certain nutrients to specified foods, and voluntary fortification, which is done by food manufacturers, in which they can add nutrients to foods as long as they follow the country's regulatory guidelines.

Are these additional micronutrients natural?

These additional micronutrients can be derived from plants or animals or created in a laboratory as synthetic chemicals.

How are fortified foods different from dietary supplements?

Both fortified foods and dietary supplements attempt to enhance the nutrition of individuals. Fortified foods contain mild vitamins and minerals, while supplements use concentrated nutrients. Fortification aims to increase the nutritional value of individuals, while supplementation works to correct any nutritional deficiencies in an individual.

Who benefits most from fortified foods?

Older people and pregnant women have higher nutritional needs, as do people who are allergic to certain foods or follow restricted diets.

How do I know if a food is fortified?

Always check the nutrition label of your packaged foods. The label will provide details about any added nutrients.

Are fortified foods safe to eat?

Fortified foods are generally safe to eat, but they shouldn't be relied upon as the sole source of nutrients. Although fortified foods may contain higher levels of some micronutrients, they cannot replace a healthy diet that includes adequate carbohydrates, protein, essential fats, and other nutrients needed for optimal health.

Consuming too many fortified foods throughout the day can also lead to nutrient overdose, especially in children. Many fortified foods available in the market contain vitamin levels that are not appropriate for children, which can be potentially dangerous.

Is fortified food good or bad?

The food industry often sells highly processed and sugary items as "fortified with essential nutrients," making people think they are making healthy choices. However, these foods are usually high in salt, trans fat, saturated fat, and sugar. Simply fortifying a food does not make it healthy. While micronutrient intake is important, healthy food should not only contain essential nutrients but also be low in sugar, salt, trans fat, and saturated fat.

Your body needs a complete diet high in whole foods, including vegetables and fruits of different colors, to stay strong and healthy.

Chapter 2
NOT TRUE VITAMINS BUT STILL VITAMINS!

Are there any vitamins other than the 13 already known?

Some compounds were previously classified as vitamins but were later either renamed to already identified vitamins or removed from the list because their health effects were not proven enough to be considered true vitamins or your body already makes these compounds in enough quantity. These vitamins that are no longer considered essential vitamins still have some positive influence on your health. These include:

Vitamin B4: Vitamin B4, also known as adenine, is a water-soluble vitamin, so it dissolves in water and should be taken daily. Adenine is a type of nucleotide found in the DNA molecule. Vitamin B4 is not classified as an essential vitamin B because your body can make adenine on its own. However, that doesn't mean it's not important; a deficiency in vitamin B4 can cause health issues. It can lower your energy levels and cause depression and neurological disorders. Adenine is found in raw honey and herbs and spices such as thyme, cloves, ginger sage, jojoba and spearmint.

Vitamin B8: Vitamin B8, also known as inositol, is a type of sugar that plays a crucial role in regulating insulin in your body. It increases insulin sensitivity in people with diabetes. It also balances certain mood-affecting neurotransmitters such as serotonin and dopamine and is beneficial in reducing anxiety, depression, and compulsive disorders. It is found in fresh and uncanned fruits, beans, grains, and nuts. Some other rich food sources of inositol are citrus fruits, cantaloupe, bran, almonds, and kidney beans.

Vitamin Bc: Vitamin Bc was reclassified as Vitamin B9 or folic acid.

Vitamin B10: Vitamin B10 is also known as para amino benzoic acid (PABA) or vitamin Bx. PABA can be synthesized by gut bacteria, which contributes to the production of some folate (or vitamin B9). Although PABA is not a true vitamin, it still has beneficial effects on your health. Low levels of PABA in your body can cause eczema and graying hair. High levels of vitamin B10 can darken gray hair, prevent sunburn, increase fertility in women, promote skin health, and reduce constipation and headaches. Some good food sources of vitamin B10 are mushrooms, spinach, brewer's yeast, sunflower seeds, milk, and wheat germ.

Vitamin B11 (Salicylic Acid): Vitamin B11 is also known as salicylic acid. Your body can synthesize salicylic acid, so the essential vitamin tag has been removed from it. Salicylic acid is great for your skin. It helps treat skin conditions. It has anti-infective and antifungal properties and when applied topically it helps remove dead cells by loosening thick and scaly skin. It softens dry skin that flakes easily. Some good food sources of vitamin B11 are broccoli, mushrooms, cucumber, cauliflower and spinach.

Peryl-hepta-glutamic acid (PHGA) was also classified as vitamin B11, but later, it was found that PHGA is a form of folate. This is why folate (vitamin B9) is also called vitamin B11 and vitamin B9.

Vitamin B13: Vitamin B13 is also known as orotic acid. Your body can synthesize orotic acid, so it is not an essential vitamin. Orotic acid is essential in the synthesis of DNA, RNA, and glycogen. It improves energy production in your body and increases resistance to ischemic stress. It is also essential in the metabolism of folate and vitamin B12. Milk, milk products, carrots, and beetroot are good sources of orotic acid.

Vitamin B14: Vitamin B14 is also known as trimethylglycine (TMG). There is much discussion about it, but it has not yet been established as a vitamin. Your body can produce trimethylglycine, which has antioxidant and anti-inflammatory properties. It enhances athletic performance and promotes heart and liver health. It also supports methylation and increases the rate of cell proliferation. Some good food sources of vitamin B14 are wheat germ, spinach, and beetroot.

Vitamin B15: Vitamin B15 is also called pangamic acid. It was promoted as a supplement that could improve stamina during exercise, improve skin conditions, and treat asthma. However, no research studies support these claims, and pangamic acid may not be safe to take orally. Some food sources of pangamic acid are yeast, apricot seeds, and corn.

Vitamin B16: Vitamin B16 is also called dimethylglycine (DMG). DMG is a derivative of an amino acid, glycine. It has a vital role in the methylation cycle and promotes energy production, enhances athletic performance, reduces lactic acid, and supports immune function. Your body can synthesize dimethylglycine as much as it needs, so it is not labeled as a vitamin. Some good sources of Vitamin B16 are beans, pumpkin seeds, brown rice, and beetroots.

Vitamin B17: It is also known as amygdalin and amygdaloside or laetrile. Amygdalin is a plant compound found in buckwheat, lima beans, millet, flaxseeds, and fruit seeds of apricots, apples, almonds, cherries, lemons, and plums. These fruits contain cyanogenic glycosides that have anti-cancer properties. However, when ingested, amygdalin reacts in the body and can cause acute cyanide infection, which causes symptoms such as confusion, anxiety, dizziness, and headaches. Laetrile is a synthetic man-made form of amygdalin that was previously used in cancer treatment but is now banned due to its toxicity.

Vitamin Bt: It is also known as carnitine or levocarnitine. Your body can make as much carnitine as it needs, so it's not a true vitamin. Carnitine helps your body convert fat into energy. Milk, avocado, asparagus, and whole wheat are good sources of carnitine.

Vitamin G: Vitamin G was reclassified as Vitamin B2 or riboflavin.

Vitamin H: Vitamin H was reclassified as Vitamin B7 or biotin.

Vitamin J: Vitamin J or flavin was similar to vitamin G and was reclassified as Vitamin B2.

Vitamin M: Vitamin M is also known as folate (in some countries as folic acid) or vitamin B9 or B11.

Vitamin PP: Vitamin Pellagra-Prevention or vitamin PP was reclassified as vitamin B3.

UNIT 2
B VITAMINS
VITAMIN B1
VITAMIN B2
VITAMIN B3
VITAMIN B5
VITAMIN B6
VITAMIN B7
VITAMIN B9
VITAMIN B12

Chapter 1
VITAMIN B1

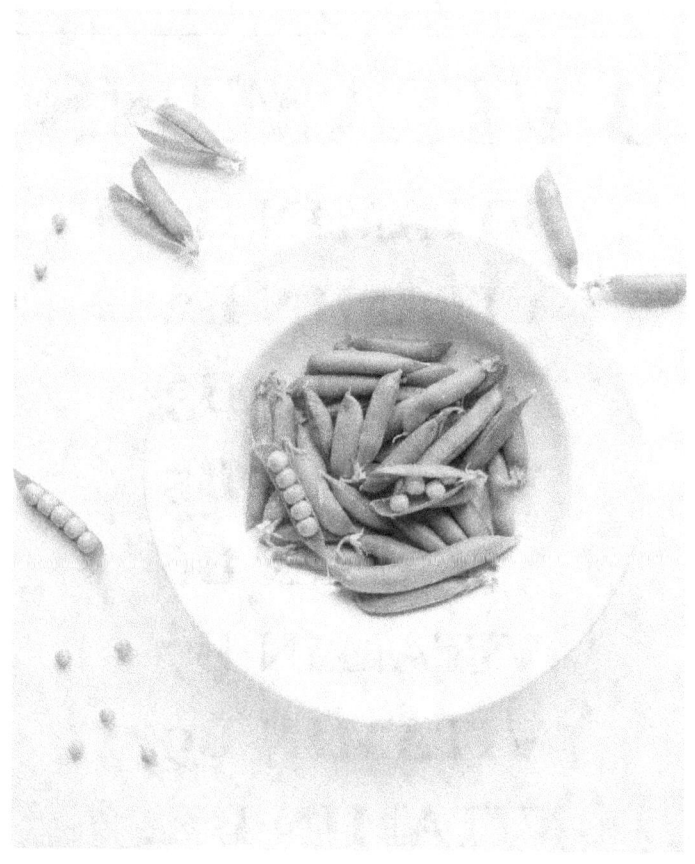

1.
EVERYTHING YOU NEED TO KNOW ABOUT VITAMIN B1

What is vitamin B1 and what does it do?

Vitamin B1, also called as thiamin (or thiamine), is an essential water-soluble vitamin required for the growth and development of the human body. Thiamin plays a critical role in the metabolism of carbohydrates, amino acids, and lipids.

How does vitamin B1 metabolize in the body?

The thiamine you consume through food is mostly (about 80%) in the phosphorylated form, and the rest is in the free form. Free thiamine is absorbed directly into the blood circulation, while the phosphorylated form needs to be released first. An enzyme called phosphatase in the intestine hydrolyses the phosphorylated thiamine and makes it free thiamine, which is then absorbed into our blood.

Is vitamin B1 stored in the body?

Unlike fat-soluble vitamins, water-soluble vitamins are stored poorly in the body. Your body stores thiamine in minimal amounts in the liver. Thiamine lasts a very short time in the body and is rapidly destroyed, so you need a constant supply from the diet.

Is vitamin B1 really an essential nutrient?

As we've learned in previous books of the 'Eat So What!' Series, essential nutrients are those that the body cannot produce on its own and must be obtained from food. Most of vitamin B1 is in the form of thiamin diphosphate (TDP) in the body. TDP is the main active form of thiamin after metabolism. It's worth noting that bacteria in the large intestine also synthesize TDP and free thiamin, but the extent of their contribution to thiamin nutrition is currently unknown. Therefore, it's essential to obtain thiamin from food to meet your body's requirements, given the current uncertainty about the role of gut bacteria.

How much vitamin B1 do I need in a day?

It's crucial to ensure that you're meeting the recommended daily intake levels of thiamin, which are sufficient to meet the nutrient requirements of healthy individuals. These levels are as follows:

Age	Male	Female
0 to 6 months*	0.2 mg	0.2 mg
7–12 months*	0.3 mg	0.3 mg
1–3 years	0.5 mg	0.5 mg
4–8 years	0.6 mg	0.6 mg
9–13 years	0.9 mg	0.9 mg
14–18 years	1.2 mg	1.0 mg
19–51+ years	1.2 mg	1.1 mg

*AI: In the absence of sufficient data to develop an RDA, the AI is an assumed intake level established to ensure nutritional adequacy.

The above data is sourced from the National Institutes of Health—Institute of Dietary Supplements.

What causes thiamine deficiency?

Poor diet: A diet that consists mainly of processed carbohydrates such as white rice, sugar, and white wheat is deficient in vitamin B1 because processing removes almost all of the vitamin B1. This can lead to vitamin B1 deficiency.

Alcohol dependence: Alcoholics often replace meals with alcohol and do not consume enough thiamine, making them prone to thiamine deficiency. In alcohol metabolism, thiamine is needed to break down ethanol into harmless byproducts. Therefore, most of the available thiamine in the body is used up in the process of alcohol metabolism, which depletes thiamine stores in the body and can lead to thiamine deficiency.

People who have diabetes: Thiamine levels in people with diabetes (particularly in type 1 diabetes) are often lower than in people who do not have diabetes. This may be due to increased clearance of thiamine by the kidneys in patients with diabetes.

Bariatric surgery: People who undergo bariatric surgery for weight loss often have malnutrition, which means that despite eating enough thiamine, it is not absorbed well in the body, which can result in thiamine deficiency. Therefore, thiamine supplementation is always recommended for patients after bariatric surgery to avoid thiamine deficiency.

Certain conditions: Certain conditions increase the body's need for thiamine, which can lead to thiamine deficiency if not met through diet. These conditions include hyperthyroidism, pregnancy, and fever.

Liver disorders: The liver, a vital organ in the body's metabolic processes, plays a crucial role in thiamine metabolism. Any disorder affecting the liver can disrupt this process, potentially leading to thiamine deficiency.

Diarrhea: Prolonged diarrhea can impair the body's absorption of thiamine, leading to a deficiency of this essential vitamin.

HIV/AIDS can decrease the absorption of vitamin B1 in the body and increase the rate of excretion of vitamin B1. As a result, less vitamin B1 is absorbed, which stays for a shorter period of time in the body, and most of the vitamin B1 is excreted through urine, which can lead to thiamin deficiency.

What are the symptoms of vitamin B1 deficiency?

The following signs and symptoms may occur in the early stages of thiamine deficiency:

- Weight loss and anorexia
- Fatigue
- muscle weakness
- Confusion
- Irritability
- Poor memory and short-term memory loss
- Sleep disturbances
- Abdominal discomfort

What happens if I am deficient in vitamin B1?

Dry beriberi: Nerve and muscle abnormalities develop in dry beriberi. It is characterized by malfunction of many peripheral nerves in the body (polyneuropathy) and muscle wasting due to thiamine deficiency. People with dry beriberi condition have impaired sensory, motor, and reflex functions. Dry beriberi mainly affects the legs, with pain in the legs, tingling in the toes, burning sensation in the legs that is particularly severe at night, and difficulty getting up from a sitting position. Persistent thiamine deficiency worsens the polyneuropathy, which may eventually affect the arms.

Wet beriberi or cardiovascular beriberi: In this condition, abnormalities develop in the heart due to thiamine deficiency. Wet beriberi causes the heart to pump more blood than normal and beat faster which results in the widening of the blood vessels, causing the skin to become hot and sweaty. The condition of beriberi is reversible, and the administration of thiamine supplements, often parenterally, quickly reverses it. However, if untreated, the heart ceases to function at this increased level for a long time, and eventually, heart failure develops. This leads to fluid accumulation in the legs (as edema) and lungs (as congestion), and blood pressure may drop, sometimes leading to shock and death.

Infantile beriberi: This form of beriberi occurs in infants who are only 3 to 4 weeks old. It occurs when the nursing mother of the baby is thiamine deficient. This can cause them to lose their voice to some extent, or they may not have certain reflexes. In infants, heart failure can occur suddenly.

Brain Abnormality:

Thiamin deficiency causes brain abnormalities, mainly in people with chronic alcoholism. It occurs about 8–10 times more commonly in people with alcohol use disorder than in general people. But this can also develop in people who have severe gastrointestinal disorders, AIDS, or drug use disorders. This brain abnormality is called the Wernicke-Korsakoff syndrome, which is a combination of two diseases, Wernicke encephalopathy and Korsakoff psychosis, and has two stages:

- **Wernicke encephalopathy:** It is an acute and life-threatening first stage in which nerves outside the brain and spinal cord are damaged, causing confusion, loss of consciousness, difficulty walking, and partial paralysis of the eyes. If left untreated, about 20% of people with Wernicke encephalopathy develop symptoms that worsen, resulting in coma and death; those who survive develop Korsakoff psychosis.

- **Korsakoff psychosis:** Although some people with Korsakoff psychosis do not already have Wernicke encephalopathy, this condition is an effect of chronic thiamine deficiency that may develop after repeated episodes of Wernicke encephalopathy. Korsakoff psychosis causes mental confusion, short-term memory loss, and confusion between real and imaginary memories, with a tendency to fabricate facts to fill in gaps in memories (a condition called confabulation).

Wernicke-Korsakoff syndrome can be treated with thiamine injections or supplements. This may improve eye condition and muscle problems. However, thiamine cannot reverse the damage already done to memory by Korsakoff syndrome.

Worsening of Diabetes Complications: People with diabetes have a greater need for thiamine than people without diabetes. Thiamine deficiency decreases insulin secretion in beta cells and impairs insulin biosynthesis. Thiamine deficiency in people with diabetes can worsen diabetes complications. Vitamin B1 plays a vital role in carbohydrate metabolism. It is also essential for the biosynthesis of nucleic acids and neurotransmitters and is a modulator of neuronal and neuromuscular transmission. In people with diabetes, thiamine deficiency in the body leads to oxidative stress, a process that causes the activation of several destructive signaling pathways. This worsens the condition of diabetic polyneuropathy, which is the malfunction of multiple peripheral nerves throughout the body.

Alzheimer's Disease: Research studies suggest that thiamine deficiency plays a role in the development of Alzheimer's disease. Some studies have found that people with cognitive impairment often have thiamine deficiency. Studies have also found that thiamine-dependent enzymes have reduced activity in the brains of people with Alzheimer's disease. This is because thiamine acts as an antioxidant in the body, and a deficiency of this vitamin causes oxidative stress in neurons, leading to the death of neurons, resulting in memory loss and plaque formation, as well as a negative impact on glucose metabolism. All of this leads to Alzheimer's disease.

What happens if I take too much thiamine?

Water-soluble vitamins are not well stored in your body. So, they don't stay in your body for long and are rapidly excreted. Thiamine is not toxic, so even if you take too much of it, it won't cause any serious adverse effects.

How is vitamin B1 deficiency diagnosed?

Initially, vitamin B1 deficiency is diagnosed based on physical examination and symptoms.

When necessary, a blood sample is collected to determine thiamine status. Thiamine status is measured by two indirect methods: assaying the activity of a particular TDP-dependent enzyme and measuring urinary thiamine excretion. Thiamin levels in the blood are not used to determine thiamin status as they are not reliable indicators of thiamin status.

The transketolase enzyme is a TDP-dependent enzyme. To determine thiamine status, the activity of the transketolase enzyme is assayed in the presence and absence of manually added TDP in ruptured red blood cells. The result reflects the extent of unsaturation of transketolase with TDP, which is known as the TDP effect.

The ranges are as follows:

0%–15%: Healthy thiamin levels

15%–25%: Marginal deficiency

> 25%: Thiamin deficiency

Another method of determining thiamine status is to measure urinary thiamine excretion. This provides data on dietary intake, but it does not show tissue stores of thiamine in the body. The ranges for urinary thiamin excretion are as follows:

More than 100 mcg/day of thiamin in urine: Sufficient thiamin intake

Less than 100 mcg/day of thiamin in urine: Insufficient thiamin intake

Less than 40 mcg/day of thiamin in urine: A deficient thiamin intake

2.
IMPORTANCE OF VITAMIN B1

FUNCTIONS OF THIAMIN IN THE BODY

Digestion of Carbohydrates

Thiamine acts as a coenzyme that is essential for the metabolism of carbohydrates, proteins, and fats. Thiamine helps convert carbohydrates into energy. The primary role of carbohydrates is to provide energy (ATP) to every cell in the body, especially in the brain and nervous system. Your body needs thiamine, which acts as a cofactor for adenosine triphosphate (ATP) production. Your body's cells need ATP to perform various functions. ATP supplies energy derived from the breakdown of food to support cellular processes such as blood circulation, muscle contractions, and body movements. Your brain is most affected by thiamine deficiency because it relies heavily on mitochondrial ATP production.

Biosynthesis of Nucleic Acids

Thiamine is involved in the biosynthesis of DNA and RNA. DNA contains the codes necessary for growth,

Nerve Signaling

Thiamine ensures the proper functioning of the central and peripheral nervous systems. It is essential for maintaining the functions of nerve membranes and supports the synthesis of myelin and several neurotransmitters, such as serotonin and acetylcholine. It is also required for the synthesis of amino acids such as aspartate and glutamate.

Like the insulation around electrical wires, myelin is an insulating sheath or layer around nerves, including brain and spinal cord nerves. The function of the myelin sheath is to speed up the transmission of electrical impulses between nerve cells. Thiamine is needed to maintain the proper structure of these myelin sheaths, contributing to the speed of nerve signaling.

Thiamine is important for brain development, function, maintenance, and the transmission of neuronal signals because enzymes involved in these processes are thiamine-dependent. These enzymes cannot function without sufficient thiamine in your body. Thiamine is involved in serotonin uptake and facilitates the GABA (γ-butyric acid) neurotransmitter uptake. A deficiency in vitamin B1 can lead to cell damage.

Thiamine as An Anti-Inflammatory Agent

Inflammation may cause tissue damage, resulting in long-term functional loss. Inflammatory cytokines such as interleukins-1 and -6 (IL-1 and IL-6) and tumor necrosis factor α (TNF-α) are rapidly released. The unbalanced production of these proinflammatory cytokines is the main reason for the reduction of membrane threshold, leading to pain and disability.

Vitamin B1 has strong anti-inflammatory effects because it inhibits the action and synthesis of inflammatory mediators. It significantly reduces the production of the proinflammatory mediators IL-1β and TNF-α. The immune system is susceptible to inflammation and oxidative stress. Vitamin B1 strengthens the immune system through its anti-inflammatory actions. It reduces stress-induced inflammation in the immune system and maintains the integrity of immune cells. They can also effectively reduce inflammation in inflammatory diseases such as arthritis.

Thiamine as An Antioxidant

When the number of free radicals in your body exceeds the antioxidants, it causes oxidative stress, which leads to cell damage. Thiamine is a powerful antioxidant, a scavenger of reactive oxygen, or a neutralizer of free radicals. Various toxic agents or byproducts of chemical processes in the body promote oxidative stress. Vitamin B1 protects against various toxic agents that cause oxidative stress and prevents the development of diseases associated with oxidative damage. Thiamine acts as a potent free radical killer and prevents oxidative stress by reducing lipid peroxidation and DNA oxidation.

Thiamine protects the immune system from oxidative damage. It prevents the stimulation of NF-κB (nuclear factor κ-light-chain-enhancer of activated B cells) caused by oxidative stress. It protects neutrophils from damage caused by oxidative stress.

Thiamine prevents the formation of advanced glycation end-products (AGEs) by non-enzymatic glycation of proteins by glucose. AGEs accompany oxidative stress and inflammation and produce free radicals (reactive oxygen). These are responsible for structural and functional modifications of proteins, cellular dysfunction, and cell death, leading to damage to tissues and organs. High levels of AGEs contribute to the development of chronic diseases such as diabetes, aging, cardiovascular diseases, and neurodegenerative diseases.

TOP HEALTH BENEFITS OF VITAMIN B1

1. **Prevent Heart Failure:** Vitamin B1 helps keep your heart healthy and prevent heart failure. The heart's energy consumption is higher than that of other organs in the body, and it requires a constant supply of

energy to function well. Vitamin B1 helps mitochondria produce energy (ATP) your heart uses to pump. Any defect in mitochondria can disrupt the normal functioning of your heart and induce cardiac dysfunction. Without enough vitamin B1, ATP production is impaired, leading to the accumulation of adenosine. This causes your heart to pump at a higher rate with increased blood volume. Over time, your heart muscle weakens, leading to a low-output state. Eventually, blood pressure drops, resulting in heart failure.

2. Boost Immunity: Vitamin B1 acts as a cofactor in the immune system. It participates in the regulation of the function of T cells, B cells, and natural killer (NK) cells. Thiamine has both anti-inflammatory and antioxidant properties. It regulates your immune response by reducing oxidative stress and inflammation, which, if not reduced, can damage immune cells and contribute to the development of various disorders. Thiamine reduces the production of inflammatory cytokines, thus protecting immune cells from inflammation. It increases the production of glutathione, a potent antioxidant. Through its antioxidant activity, thiamine protects immune cells from the negative effects of oxidative stress by neutralizing free radicals.

3. Anti-Stress Vitamin: Thiamine is sometimes also referred as the anti-stress vitamin. It is effective in treating a variety of anxiety disorders. It is considered a protective vitamin for the adrenal gland. The adrenal glands (on top of your kidneys) release the stress hormone cortisol, which has an essential role in the body's response to stressful situations. Thiamine enhances the positive stress response and may reduce the stress-induced cortisol response. Additionally, it helps treat anxiety by keeping your nervous system healthy, which is necessary to combat the high-stress levels that accompany anxiety.

4. Supports Your Nervous System: B vitamins, especially thiamine (B1), pyridoxine (B6), and cobalamin (B12), are the main vitamins for maintaining neuronal viability. Vitamin B1, together with B6 and B12, protects nerves from the harmful effects of the environment. Vitamin B1 is a powerful antioxidant, vitamin B6 regulates nerve metabolism, and vitamin B12 maintains the myelin sheath. Vitamins B1, B6, and B12 support the growth of new cell structures and are important for the regeneration of cells. Vitamin B1 facilitates the use of carbohydrates for energy production, while vitamin B12 enhances nerve cell survival and speeds up the transmission of signals between neurons. Low levels of vitamins B1, B6, and B12 can cause permanent nerve degeneration and pain, eventually leading to nerve damage.

Thiamine deficiency affects your peripheral nerves. These nerves are responsible for sending signals to your brain to help with balance and coordination. They are also responsible for making you feel hot and cold sensation.

5. Prevent Cataract Development: High intake of vitamin B1 along with protein, vitamin A, vitamins B2, B3, B9, and B12 is associated with a lower prevalence of cataracts. These eye nutrients protect the lens of your eyes from developing cataracts. Cataracts and other eye disorders develop due to the toxic effects of free radicals produced through energy production, nutrient metabolism, and external factors such as pollution, ultraviolet light, and radioactive radiation. Vitamin B1 kills free radicals through its antioxidant properties. Thiamine prevents cell damage caused by free radicals and protects the lens of your eyes from developing cataracts and other eye disorders.

6. Prevent Alzheimer's Disease: Thiamine can protect you from developing Alzheimer's disease. There are several ways through which it prevents Alzheimer's disease. Thiamine acts as an antioxidant and protects your neurons from damage caused by oxidative stress, which, if not controlled, can lead to the death of neurons and memory loss. It prevents the build-up of proteins in your brain, which, if not prevented, can form plaques in your brain, causing brain cells to die. Vitamin B1 is essential for glucose metabolism. Its deficiency reduces the activity of the thiamine-dependent enzyme transketolase in your brain, leading to Alzheimer's disease.

7. Maintain Mental Health: Your brain is the most energy-demanding organ due to its complex neurons or nerve cells. Your brain uses 20 percent of the body's total energy production, which is more than any other organ. Mental health issues like depression, insomnia, confusion, and anxiety occur when your brain does not get the required amount and constant supply of energy. Vitamin B1 helps the mitochondria in brain cells to convert glucose from the carbohydrates you eat through food into energy. Vitamin B1 ensures a constant energy supply to the brain and keeps the brain cells healthy, which prevents mental health problems as well as helps your body cope with high-stress situations.

8. Better Blood Sugar Management: People with type-1 and type-2 diabetes often have low thiamine levels. Adding more vitamin B1 to your diet can help you manage your blood sugar levels. Thiamine acts as an antioxidant and prevents oxidative stress; it accelerates glucose metabolism and eliminates toxic metabolites. These metabolites accumulate in thiamine deficiency, and excess accumulation of these can lead to the development of diabetes in the long term. Also, thiamine is essential for the synthesis of insulin and its release in beta cells, which helps keep your blood sugar levels normal.

High blood glucose levels can injure nerves throughout the body. One of the common complications of diabetes is diabetic neuropathy. This is characterised by nerve damage that causes pain and numbness primarily in the legs and feet due to high blood sugar levels. Thiamine improves nerve health and may reduce pain associated with diabetic neuropathy.

3.
10 RICHEST VEGETARIAN SOURCES OF VITAMIN B1

Below are the 10 richest vegetarian sources of Vitamin B1 (Thiamine):

1. Dry Yeast/Baker's Yeast

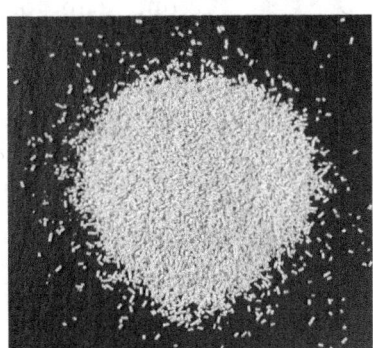

Dry yeast is a great way to add thiamine to your diet while enjoying homemade multigrain bread or whole wheat pizzas. One packet (7 g) of active dry yeast contains 66% of your daily requirement of thiamine. Using whole wheat flour when making bread or pizza can give you more than 100% of your daily requirement of thiamine, as whole wheat also contains a good amount of thiamine.

2. Beans and Lentils

Beans and lentils are the richest sources of vitamin B1. They provide not only vitamin B1 but also protein, minerals, and fiber. One cup of cooked soybeans contains 39% of the daily requirement of thiamine, one cup of cooked black beans contains 35% of the daily

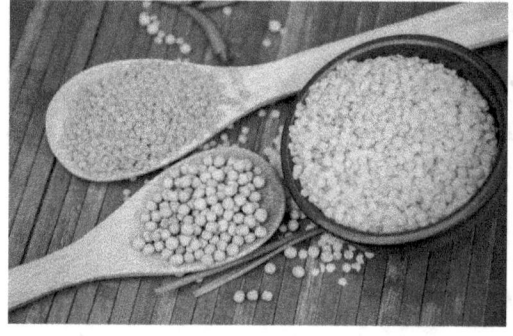

requirement of thiamine, one cup of cooked mung beans contains 28% daily value of thiamine, one cup of cooked lentils contains 28% DV of thiamine, one cup of cooked kidney beans contains 24% DV of thiamine and one cup of cooked chickpeas contains 16% of the daily requirement of thiamine.

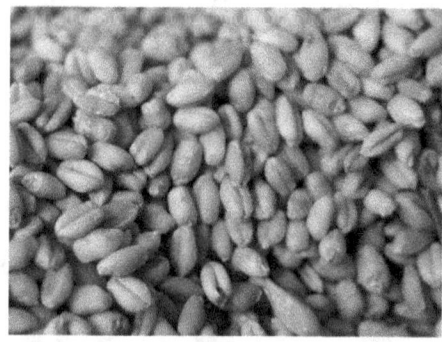

3. Whole Grains

Whole grains such as brown rice, whole grain chapattis, and multigrain bread are some of the best vegetarian sources of thiamine. They can fulfill up to 47% of your daily requirement of vitamin

B1. Whole grain foods have zero cholesterol, which helps control cholesterol levels and blood pressure, and are weight-friendly. These foods also help reduce the risk of diabetes, heart disease, and other chronic diseases.

4. Green Peas

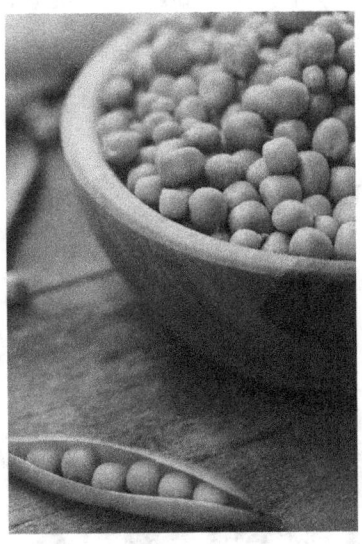

Green peas are a great vegetarian source of vitamin B1. 100 g of green peas contain 0.282 mg of vitamin B1, equivalent to 25% of the daily thiamine requirement. They are also high in protein, fiber, and minerals like iron, potassium, magnesium, and selenium. They are also rich in antioxidants that boost immune health.

5. Sunflower Seeds

Sunflower seeds can provide some of the thiamine you need for the day. Half a cup of roasted sunflower seeds can meet 25% of the daily requirement of thiamine. Not only thiamine, they contain a good amount of fiber and are also a great source of fat-soluble vitamins like vitamin E. Sunflower seeds are high in beneficial

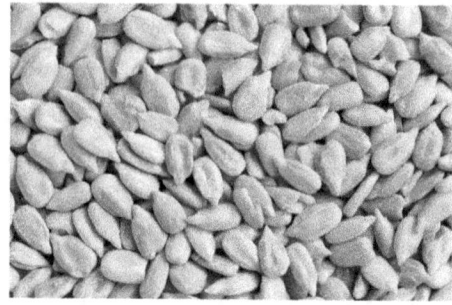

polyunsaturated fats that are anti-inflammatory and good for the heart when eaten in moderation. Additionally, sunflower seeds are also packed with selenium, zinc, folate, and protein.

6. Flax Seeds

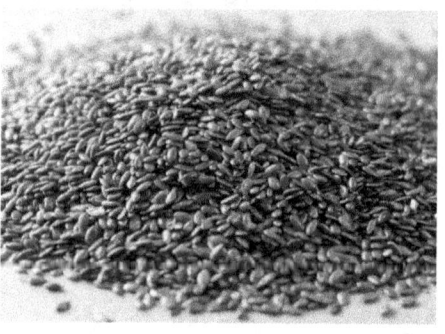

You may know that flax seeds are an excellent source of omega-3 fats, but they are also a good source of thiamine. One tablespoon of whole flax seeds can give you 15% of your daily thiamine requirement. Use ground flax seeds instead of whole flax seeds, as ground flax seeds are easier to digest. Make sure to drink a glass of water after consuming flax seeds, as they have a tendency to swell, and they may draw water from your body to swell if you have insufficient water intake.

7. Oats

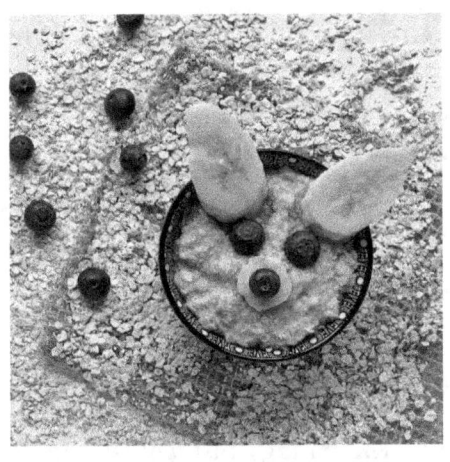

Oats are a great source of manganese and soluble fiber and also a great source of vitamin B1. 100 g of oats contains 64% of the daily requirement of thiamine. Daily consumption of oats can reduce bad LDL cholesterol and blood sugar, thereby reducing the risk of heart disease. The high amount of manganese and thiamine in oats helps control blood sugar levels and promote healthy brain and nerve function.

8. Milk

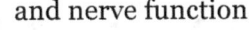

Milk can fulfill some of the thiamine requirements in a day. 1 cup of milk can give you 12% of the daily thiamine requirement. Milk is considered a complete food as it has almost all the nutrients the human body requires. So, milk provides you with all the vitamins, minerals, proteins, and fats required daily, along with the necessary thiamine.

9. Pistachios

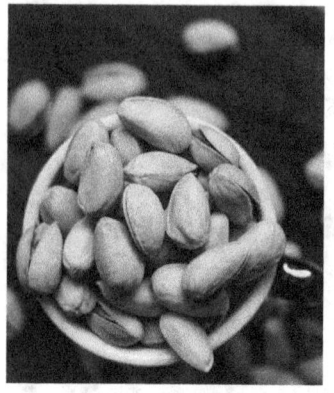

Pistachios are not just a tasty snack; they can also meet your daily thiamine requirement. Compared to other nuts, pistachios are lower in fat and are primarily composed of good fats. They are also a great source of protein, fiber, vitamin B6, vitamin E, and K. Eating pistachios can prevent baldness, especially in men. A mere handful of pistachios (30 grams) contain 22% of your daily thiamine requirement, making them a unique and intriguing addition to your diet.

10. Acorn Squash

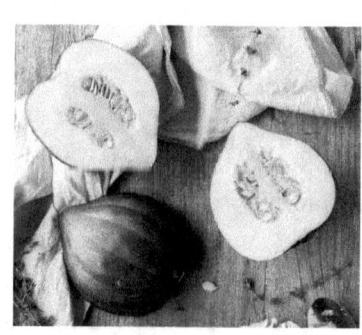

Acorn squash is a fair source of thiamine and vitamin C. 1 cup of baked acorn squash can meet 34% of your daily requirement of vitamin B1. Its thiamine content not only supports nerve health and muscle mass but also enhances heart function. It enhances your memory and helps improve concentration. The high antioxidant content of squash can boost the health of your immune system and strengthen your bones and blood vessels.

Chapter 2
VITAMIN B2

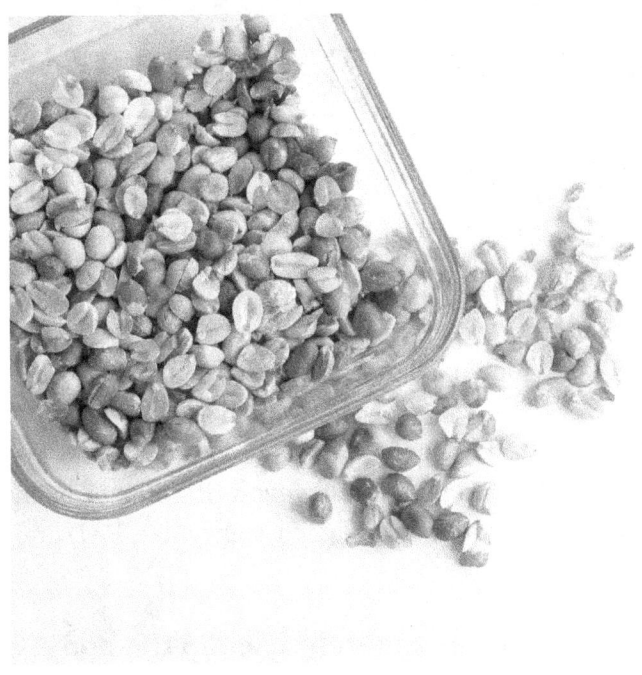

1.
EVERYTHING YOU NEED TO KNOW ABOUT VITAMIN B2

What is vitamin B2, and what does it do?

Our next B vitamin is riboflavin, also known as vitamin B2. Two important coenzymes, flavin mononucleotide (FMN) and flavin adenine dinucleotide (FAD) play vital roles in the body. They are necessary for the metabolism of carbohydrates to produce energy, normal bodily function, and growth. Riboflavin is an essential component of these two coenzymes, FAD and FAM.

How is vitamin B2 metabolized in the body?

More than 90% of the riboflavin in your food is in the form of FAD or FMN (also called riboflavin-5'-phosphate), with only 10% in the free form. Riboflavin is absorbed primarily in your small intestine. Riboflavin from foods is better absorbed than vitamin supplements in your body. It is important to consume riboflavin daily through food because your body only absorbs about 15% of it, and the rest is excreted in urine.

Is vitamin B2 stored in the body?

Like other water-soluble vitamins, riboflavin is stored in very small amounts in the liver, heart, and kidneys. Consuming too much riboflavin may either not be absorbed at all, or the little that is absorbed is quickly excreted through urine.

Is vitamin B6 really an essential nutrient?

The free form of riboflavin can be produced by bacteria in your large intestine, which can be absorbed by your body, but the amount produced is not enough to meet dietary requirements, so you have to eat riboflavin-rich foods every day to meet your body's requirements. Interestingly, the bacteria in the large intestine produce more riboflavin after consuming vegetable-based meals than meat-based foods.

How much vitamin B2 do I need a day?

The recommended daily level of riboflavin intake sufficient to meet the vitamin B2 requirements of healthy people is as follows:

Age	Male	Female
Birth to 6	0.3 mg	0.3 mg
7–12 m	0.4 mg	0.4 mg
1–3 yrs.	0.5 mg	0.5 mg

4–8 yrs.	0.6 mg	0.6 mg
9–13 yrs.	0.9 mg	0.9 mg
14–18 yrs.	1.3 mg	1.0 mg
19+ yrs.	1.3 mg	1.1 mg

*AI: In the absence of sufficient data to develop an RDA, Adequate Intake (AI) is considered, which is the intake level estimated to ensure nutritional adequacy.

What are the symptoms of riboflavin deficiency?

Riboflavin deficiency is also known as ariboflavinosis. Some common symptoms are given below:

- Painful cracks at the corners of the mouth
- Swollen and cracked lips.
- Pale skin.
- Sore mouth, tongue, and throat.
- Itchy and red eyes.
- Tongue and mouth may turn magenta.
- Excess blood in vessels.
- Hair loss.
- Seborrheic red and scaly patches around the nose, on the ears and eyebrows, between the nose and the lips, and in the genital area.
- Cataract formation due to prolonged riboflavin deficiency.

People who are deficient in riboflavin usually also have deficiencies in other nutrients. This is because severe riboflavin deficiency can lower flavin coenzyme levels, which impairs the metabolism of other B vitamins.

Riboflavin deficiency can be easily corrected with vitamin supplements. However, riboflavin supplements cannot reverse the damage that has already occurred, such as cataract formation, due to long-term riboflavin deficiency.

What if I am deficient in vitamin B2?

Vitamin B2 is essential for the body to produce energy and for cellular function. Vitamin B2 deficiency interferes with the normal functioning of the body and may lead to the following diseases:

Anemia: Riboflavin increases your body's absorption of iron. Iron is required to make hemoglobin, a protein present in red blood cells (RBCs) that transports oxygen to cells. Riboflavin deficiency alters iron absorption and reduces the release of iron from stores, leading to iron deficiency and anemia.

Migraine: Mitochondria are present in almost every cell in your body. Its main function is to produce energy (ATP) needed to power the cells to perform bodily functions. Riboflavin is an important component of mitochondrial energy production. Riboflavin is involved in carbohydrate metabolism and is particularly essential for the normal production of ATP (the energy currency of the cell). In an adult brain, neurons have the highest demand for energy.

Carbohydrates are the brain's main source of energy and require a consistent supply of glucose from the blood. Riboflavin deficiency can lead to mitochondrial dysfunction. Any impairment of mitochondria in the brain ultimately leads to a decrease in mitochondrial energy and can cause migraines.

Cataract and other eye disorders: Riboflavin deficiency is directly linked to cataract formation and other eye disorders like glaucoma and keratoconus. Riboflavin participates in the glutathione redox reaction involving glutathione reductase, which is an FAD-dependent enzyme. Glutathione (GSH) is an organic compound with antioxidant properties that kills harmful free radicals but becomes inactive during the process. The FAD-dependent enzyme glutathione reductase enzyme can reactivate oxidized glutathione back to glutathione. Long-term riboflavin deficiency plays an important role in causing cataracts because riboflavin is involved in the regeneration of reduced GSH during the redox reaction.

Liver degeneration: Riboflavin is found in high concentrations in the liver and kidney. Liver degeneration is expected to occur with riboflavin deficiency. Riboflavin deficiency leads to the accumulation of lipids in the liver and increases the concentration of saturated fatty acids (SFA). This leads to proinflammatory responses that can cause liver hypertrophy.

Other B Vitamin Deficiencies: Riboflavin deficiency impairs the metabolism of other nutrients, especially the B vitamins. The riboflavin derivative FAD or FMN is required for the synthesis of vitamin B3 and the metabolism of vitamins B6, B12, folate, and iron. FAD is essential for folate metabolism, acting as a cofactor for an important folate-metabolizing enzyme. The conversion of vitamin B6 (pyridoxine) to its active coenzyme form requires the enzyme pyridoxine 5'-phosphate oxidase (PPO), an FMN-dependent enzyme.

Tryptophan is an amino acid converted into NAD and NADP coenzymes containing niacin or vitamin B3. The conversion of tryptophan to NAD and NADP requires an FAD-dependent enzyme, kynurenine 3-monooxygenase.

Riboflavin is also essential for folate metabolism, where the riboflavin derivative FAD is required as a cofactor for a major folate-metabolizing enzyme, methylenetetrahydrofolate reductase (MTHFR). Riboflavin is a determinant of homocysteine levels in the body. Homocysteine (an amino acid) comes from the breakdown of methionine, an essential amino acid used for protein synthesis. Methylenetetrahydrofolate reductase (MTHFR) is a FAD-dependent enzyme that helps break down homocysteine. Homocysteine can be reconverted to methionine by methionine synthase with the help of folate coenzymes and methylcobalamin, the active form of vitamin B12. Both riboflavin derivatives, FAD and FMN, act as coenzymes for the methionine synthase reductase enzyme. This enzyme regenerates methylcobalamin, which acts as a coenzyme for methionine synthase. Riboflavin deficiency can disrupt these processes and result in high levels of homocysteine in the body, leading to cardiovascular disorders.

Severe riboflavin deficiency may decrease niacin synthesis and conversion of vitamin B6 to its active form, impair folate metabolism, and increase homocysteine levels.

Development of cardiovascular diseases: Riboflavin deficiency is associated with high levels of plasma homocysteine, an amino acid in the blood, which is associated with a higher risk of cardiovascular disease, stroke, dementia, and other chronic diseases—vitamins B6, B12, and folic acid break down homocysteine into other substances that your body needs. Since riboflavin is involved in the metabolism of vitamins B6, B12, and folate, its deficiency leads to vitamin B6, B12, and folate deficiency. Without these three vitamins, homocysteine remains high in your blood, which eventually leads to chronic diseases.

Poor skin and hair health: Collagen is a protein found primarily in your skin, hair, and nails. Riboflavin is essential for the synthesis of collagen. Riboflavin deficiency reduces collagen levels, resulting in weak nails, brittle hair, and dry skin.

Alzheimer's Disease and Parkinson's Disease: Riboflavin has antioxidant properties. Riboflavin deficiency leads to the oxidation of proteins and DNA strands. As a result, the tissue loses its ability to restore itself, and DNA gets damaged. Riboflavin deficiency means low antioxidant activity in the body, which increases the activity of free radicals, resulting in the accumulation of proteins with incorrect structure. This leads to misfolded proteins, which contribute to the development of Alzheimer's, Huntington's, and Parkinson's disease.

What causes riboflavin deficiency?

Vitamin B2 deficiency is primarily caused by a poor diet that lacks vitamin B2. Secondary riboflavin deficiency occurs when vitamin B2 is not absorbed by the intestine or, your body is unable to use it, or it may be excreted too quickly through urine. Below are conditions that interfere with the absorption, use, or excretion of vitamin B2, leading to vitamin B2 deficiency:

Poor diet: Lack of vitamin B2-rich foods like milk and almonds can lead to vitamin B2 deficiency.

Certain disorders: Diarrhea, liver disorders, and alcohol consumption interfere with the absorption of vitamin B2 in your body as well as increase its excretion through urine. This can lead to riboflavin deficiency.

Certain medications: Excessive use of antianxiety and sedative drugs like barbiturates can reduce riboflavin levels in your body.

Malabsorption syndromes: Certain conditions, such as short bowel syndrome and celiac disease, prevent your body's absorption of vitamin B2, even if you eat enough. Malabsorption can cause vitamin B2 deficiency.

Thyroid hormone deficiency: Riboflavin in your body is converted to riboflavin mononucleotide and then to its active coenzyme form, flavin adenine dinucleotide (FAD). This conversion is controlled by thyroid hormone. The thyroxine (T4) hormone is required for the riboflavin to flavin adenine dinucleotide (FAD) conversion. Hypothyroidism reduces FAD levels to levels seen in riboflavin deficiency.

Who is prone to riboflavin deficiency?

Athletes: Excessive exercise can reduce riboflavin levels due to the stress produced by exercise in metabolic pathways. They have an increased need for riboflavin, which, if not met, can lead to a deficiency of this vitamin.

Older people: As you age, your need for riboflavin increases due to a decrease in the body's absorption of riboflavin. This increased requirement is often not met by diet and puts you at risk for riboflavin deficiency.

Pregnancy: Pregnancy requires a higher intake of riboflavin. The baby will likely have a riboflavin deficiency if the mother has low riboflavin levels during pregnancy. This is why pregnant women are often given riboflavin supplements.

Lactose intolerant: Milk and milk products are excellent sources of vitamin B2. Due to a low intake of milk products, people with lactose intolerance often have low levels of riboflavin.

Is riboflavin sensitive to light?

Riboflavin is highly sensitive to light. Exposure to ultraviolet or even visible light can rapidly inactivate riboflavin and its derivatives. Because of the loss of riboflavin in the presence of light, milk is not typically stored in glass containers. Any riboflavin-containing food stored in a glass container exposed to light contains less riboflavin than foods not exposed to light.

What happens if I take too much riboflavin?

Water-soluble vitamins are not stored in the body. So they don't stay in your system for long and are readily excreted. There have been no known side effects from consuming too much riboflavin through food. Riboflavin is not toxic, so even if you take too much of it, it won't cause serious adverse effects. However, be cautious about taking too much riboflavin through supplements. Just because data on adverse effects is limited does not mean that a high intake of riboflavin does not cause any adverse effects.

How is riboflavin deficiency diagnosed?

How is riboflavin deficiency diagnosed? Riboflavin deficiency is diagnosed based on typical symptoms such as painful cracks in the corners of the mouth and magenta discoloration of the tongue. The deficiency is confirmed in two ways:

Blood Test

A simple blood sample is collected to measure riboflavin status. Vitamin B2 is a component of the flavin adenine dinucleotide (FAD) co-enzyme. The erythrocyte glutathione reductase activity coefficient (EGRAC) is a common test to measure riboflavin deficiency. In this, the activity of an FAD-dependent enzyme called erythrocyte glutathione reductase (EGR) is assayed in the presence and absence of added FAD. The ratio between the activities of this enzyme in the presence of FAD and without FAD indicates riboflavin status. The limits are given below:

1.2 or less − Adequate riboflavin status

1.2–1.4 = Marginal deficiency

More than 1.4 = Riboflavin deficiency

Urine Test

Another method of determining riboflavin status is the fluorometric measurement of urinary excretion over 24 hours. It is expressed as the total amount of riboflavin excreted. It provides data on dietary intake, but it does not show tissue stores of riboflavin. Urine excretion measurement is less accurate than EGRAC. Various factors can affect urinary excretion levels, such as in stressful situations, and with certain medications, urine may increase or decrease with age. In addition, the amount excreted mainly reflects recent riboflavin intake, not long-term riboflavin status.

Total riboflavin excretion ranges are as follows:

At least 120 mcg/day = Normal

A rate of less than 40 mcg/day = Riboflavin deficiency

2. IMPORTANCE OF VITAMIN B2

FUNCTIONS OF RIBOFLAVIN IN THE BODY

Energy Production

Vitamin B2 is essential for the body's growth and development. Carbohydrates, fats, and proteins from your diet are metabolized into glucose. Your body needs vitamin B2 to convert food into energy (ATP production), which is used to fuel every cell to perform bodily functions. The coenzyme forms of riboflavin (vitamin B2), flavin adenine dinucleotide (FAD), and flavin mononucleotide (FMN) serve as electron carriers that play a vital role in the generation of ATP (the energy currency of cells).

Red Blood Cell Production

Riboflavin increases hemoglobin levels and red blood cell count in the body. Hemoglobin is a protein found in red blood cells. It gives blood cells their red color and is responsible for delivering oxygen to every tissue in the body. Iron is essential for hemoglobin production. Without enough iron, your body cannot produce hemoglobin. Iron is not absorbed well in the body; without absorption, you do not get the benefits of iron even if you consume enough iron through food. Vitamin B2 increases iron absorption in the body. It also helps mobilize iron from stores when needed. Better absorption of iron results in the formation of more hemoglobin, which in turn increases red blood cell production.

Synthesis of Vitamin B3

Vitamin B2 acts as a coenzyme in vitamin B3 synthesis. Tryptophan is an amino acid that is converted into the coenzymes nicotinamide adenine dinucleotide phosphate (NADP) and nicotinamide adenine dinucleotide (NAD). Both of these coenzymes comprise vitamin B3 or niacin. The conversion of tryptophan into niacin containing NAD and NADP requires the kynurenine 3-monooxygenase enzyme, which needs the vitamin B2 derivative, flavin adenine dinucleotide (FAD), to function. Without enough vitamin B2 in your body, it cannot make enough vitamin B3; a vitamin B2 deficiency can lead to vitamin B3 deficiency.

Converting Vitamin B6 to Its Active Form

The vitamin is usually inactive, which means your body cannot absorb it in this form. Your liver converts the vitamin into its active form, which the body can then absorb and use. Vitamin B6 must be converted into its active coenzyme form, pyridoxal 5'-phosphate (PLP) to perform its action. This conversion is catalyzed by an FMN-dependent enzyme called pyridoxine 5'-phosphate oxidase (PPO). Vitamin B2 deficiency affects the levels of active vitamin B6 in your body. The importance of this relationship in maintaining vitamin B6 status is not yet scientifically clear, but it can certainly affect vitamin B6 levels in the body to some extent.

Regulates Homocysteine Levels

Homocysteine is an amino acid derived from the breakdown of methionine, an essential amino acid used for protein synthesis. High homocysteine levels in the body can cause cardiovascular disorders, so the breakdown of homocysteine is important for preventing cardiovascular disease and other chronic diseases. Homocysteine can be converted back to methionine.

Methylenetetrahydrofolate reductase (MTHFR) plays a critical role in the breakdown of homocysteine. It catalyzes the formation of 5-methyltetrahydrofolate, the primary coenzyme form of folate used to convert homocysteine to methionine. This MTHFR is a FAD-dependent enzyme. Riboflavin-derived FAD serves as a cofactor for MTHFR.

Homocysteine is reconverted into methionine by methionine synthase with the help of the folate coenzyme 5-methyl THF and methylcobalamin, the active form of vitamin B12. Methionine synthase reductase (MTRR) acts as a coenzyme for methionine synthase, which regenerates methylcobalamin into active form so that it can participate in remethylation again. Methionine synthase reductase is a riboflavin-dependent enzyme. Both riboflavin derivatives, FAD and FMN, act as coenzymes for the enzyme methionine synthase reductase.

Riboflavin deficiency affects the body's levels of methylenetetrahydrofolate reductase (MTHFR) and methionine synthase reductase (MTRR). Low MTHFR and MTRR levels inhibit the conversion of homocysteine to methionine, which increases the homocysteine levels in the body and increases the risk of heart disease, stroke, and dementia.

Riboflavin as An Antioxidant

Riboflavin indirectly exerts antioxidant action; it regenerates glutathione, a free radical scavenger. Aerobic respiration is a process in which oxygen is utilized to make energy from carbohydrates (glucose). Aerobic respiration is also called cell respiration or oxidative metabolism. This process produces free radicals, which are inactivated by antioxidant defense systems. However, oxidative stress results from an imbalance between the generation of free radicals in the body and the ability of antioxidant defense mechanisms to inactivate them. Free radicals can also be formed due to external factors like stress, pollution, and UV rays. The imbalance or oxidative stress is involved in the development of many chronic diseases, such as diabetes, heart disease, cancer, and some neurodegenerative diseases. Although riboflavin has a pro-oxidant effect when exposed to ultraviolet radiation, several studies have proven its antioxidant potential.

Aerobic respiration involves several reactions involving electron transfer and are known as redox reactions or oxidation-reduction reactions. Glutathione (GSH) is a powerful antioxidant and a major detoxification agent in cells. The glutathione redox cycle protects cells by neutralizing free radicals or reactive oxygen species. However, during this process, it gets oxidized and inactivated. Glutathione reductase (GR) is an FAD-dependent enzyme that participates in the redox cycle of glutathione. Glutathione reductase is responsible for converting oxidized glutathione back to its reduced form (active form). Once reactivated, it can perform its function again and kill free radicals.

TOP HEALTH BENEFITS OF VITAMIN B2

1. Prevent Migraine: Riboflavin is involved in carbohydrate metabolism and is particularly essential for the normal production of ATP. Mitochondria are organelles that convert energy derived from glucose into adenosine triphosphate (ATP). ATP is the energy currency that cells need to function. Riboflavin derivatives flavin mononucleotide (FMN) and flavin adenine dinucleotide (FAD) act as enzymatic cofactors and participate in several energy metabolism mechanisms. Your brain has the highest energy demand. Riboflavin deficiency can lead to mitochondrial dysfunction. Any defect in the brain's mitochondria leads to a deficit in mitochondrial energy, which may cause migraines. Eating enough riboflavin-rich foods prevents migraine by ensuring continuous glucose delivery through the blood to the brain.

2. Prevent Anemia: Anemia is a condition that occurs when your blood contains fewer healthy red blood cells than normal. A low RBC count causes you to feel tired and exhausted because your body does not get enough oxygen-rich blood. Riboflavins are involved in producing red blood cells (RBCs) and transporting oxygen to the tissues in the body. Riboflavin enhances iron absorption and increases the mobilization of iron from stores. Iron is needed to form hemoglobin, a main component in red blood cells that enables them to carry oxygen. Eating enough riboflavin-rich foods can increase hemoglobin levels in your body, boost red blood cell production, and prevent anemia.

3. Healthy Hair: Vitamin B2 plays a vital role in increasing hemoglobin and the production of red blood cells. It increases the absorption of iron in your body. More RBCs mean more oxygen and vital nutrients that reach your hair follicles and promote hair growth.

Vitamin B2 is essential for thyroid hormone synthesis, and its antioxidant property protects the thyroid gland from oxidative stress. Thyroid hormones are important for the growth and maintenance of healthy hair. Maintaining optimal thyroid hormone levels promotes hair growth and hair health.

Additionally, vitamin B2 is involved in the synthesis of collagen, which is the primary structural protein found in hair. Collagen provides elasticity and strength to your hair. It helps reduce split ends, dry hair, and frizzy hair. Vitamin B2 is essential for maintaining adequate levels of collagen in the body. A deficiency of vitamin B2 can lead to hair breakage, split ends, and dry hair.

4. Healthy Skin: Collagen is a protein essential for skin elasticity and firmness that is primarily found in your skin. Low collagen levels can cause dry and aged skin. Riboflavin is essential for the synthesis of collagen and maintaining its adequate levels in the body. High collagen levels aid in tissue repair and help prevent wrinkles, sagging, and aged skin. Riboflavin is responsible for skin elasticity and firmness.

5. Prevent Cataracts and Other Eye Disorders: Research has shown that adequate riboflavin-rich foods reduce the risk of eye disorders. Cataracts and other eye diseases can develop from severe and long-term riboflavin deficiency. Riboflavin prevents blurred vision by protecting the eye lens and may help prevent cataracts. Glutathione reductase is an enzyme that participates in the glutathione redox cycle, and it requires the riboflavin derivative FAD to perform its action. Redox reactions produce energy (ATP) for cells. Glutathione is an antioxidant that protects cells by killing free radicals, but it gets oxidized in the process and needs to be regenerated to kill more free radicals. The glutathione reductase enzyme can regenerate oxidized glutathione. Since glutathione reductase is a FAD-dependent enzyme, in the scenario of riboflavin deficiency, it cannot perform its action, resulting in increased oxidative stress leading to cataracts and other eye disorders. The involvement of riboflavin in the regeneration of reduced glutathione plays an essential role in protecting against cataract development.

Riboflavin also acts as a photosensitizer to treat certain eye disorders. Riboflavin drops are usually applied to the corneal surface for treating corneal ectasia eye disorders. Riboflavin is light sensitive, and under ultraviolet light, it acts as a prooxidant and increases the production of free radicals that induce cross-linking of corneal collagen. Increasing the cross-linking of corneal collagen increases the stiffness and strength of the cornea.

6. Prevent Coronary Heart Disease and Stroke: Vitamin B2 helps prevent coronary heart disease, stroke, and other chronic diseases as it is essential for maintaining normal levels of homocysteine in your body. Vitamin B2 works with other B vitamins, B6, B12, and folate, to maintain low homocysteine concentrations in your blood. Homocysteine is formed by the breakdown of the essential amino acid methionine. Methionine is the building block used to make proteins and is important for cell and DNA function. When it breaks down into homocysteine, it becomes a harmful agent that increases the risk of coronary heart disease and stroke. Vitamin B2 ensures that homocysteine is converted back to methionine and reduces homocysteine levels. Lower homocysteine helps lower blood pressure and reduces your risk of heart disease and stroke by 25%.

7. Cancer Prevention and Treatment: Consuming adequate amounts of riboflavin can help you prevent cancer. Riboflavin participates in the metabolism of other nutrients and is a determinant of homocysteine levels in your body. In addition, riboflavin is a potent antioxidant and prevents DNA damage caused by several carcinogens. These collective actions of riboflavin help prevent various types of cancer.

New research has shown that vitamin B2 can inhibit the growth and spread of cancer cells. Cancer stem cells cause tumors. Energy-producing mitochondria are found in every cell, even cancer cells. Mitochondria provide energy for every cell to function, but it helps them grow and spread in cancer cells. As discussed above, vitamin B2 is essential in mitochondria energy production. Inhibition of cancer cell proliferation by vitamin B2 is achieved by blocking vitamin B2 in cancer cells. As a result, mitochondria in cancer cells cannot produce enough energy to survive, and cancer cells die due to lack of energy.

8. Maintain Thyroid Function: Vitamin B2 affects thyroid function. Vitamin B2 is essential for the synthesis of thyroid hormones. Riboflavin-derived FAD is required for the organification of iodine (a process in which iodine is incorporated into thyroglobulin to produce thyroid hormones). Vitamin B2 also aids in the conversion of T4 (thyroxine) to the active form T3 (triiodothyronine). T4 to T3 conversion is essential for controlling your body metabolism, stimulating your nervous system, regulating body temperature, and properly functioning your organs. T4 to T3 conversion significantly reduces iron deficiency in your body.

In addition, high rates of hormone production and iodine use can produce free radicals and make the thyroid prone to oxidative damage. Riboflavin is a potent antioxidant; it protects the thyroid gland from oxidative stress and maintains its health and functionality.

3.
10 RICHEST VEGETARIAN SOURCES OF VITAMIN B2

Below are the 10 richest vegetarian sources of Vitamin B2 (Riboflavin):

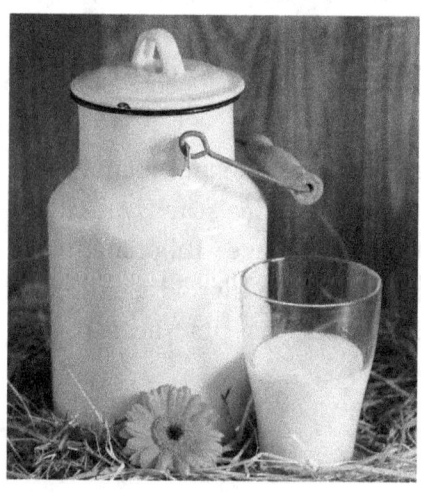

1. Milk

Milk is an excellent source of Riboflavin. Along with vitamin B2, it also provides vitamin B12 and vitamin D. All these vitamins produce synergistic effects and promote overall health. They increase energy levels, and promote bone, immune system, eye, and brain health. One cup (250 ml) of milk can help you prevent various vitamin deficiencies. As far as riboflavin is concerned,

1 cup of low-fat milk provides 38% of the riboflavin your body needs in a day.

2. Milk Products

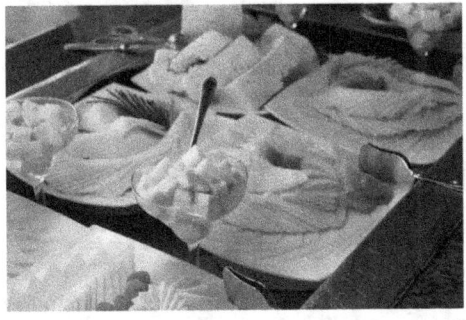

Milk products are great sources of vitamin B2. They are not only rich in vitamin B2 but also contain other essential vitamins and minerals. Yogurt is rich in vitamin B2 and is also great for your digestive system and bones. They also help maintain a healthy weight. 1 cup of yogurt can meet 46% of your daily vitamin B2 requirement. Other milk products that are high in vitamin B2 are buttermilk; 1 cup of buttermilk contains 32% of the daily requirement of vitamin B2 and homemade cottage cheese; 100 grams of cottage cheese contains 20% of the daily requirement of vitamin B2.

3. Almonds

When you think of improving memory, almonds come to mind. Even when you think of healthy skin and hair, almonds come to mind. Almonds are loaded with various health benefits. This tree nut contains more vitamin B2, vitamin E, and calcium than any other nut. Being rich in healthy fats, almonds lower cholesterol levels, regulate blood pressure, and keep your heart healthy. Vitamin B2 in

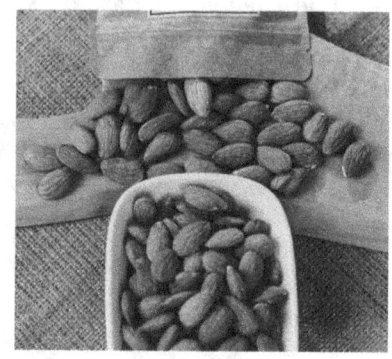

almonds prevents eye disorders, improves muscle strength, and prevents brain defects. A handful of dry-roasted almonds contains 23% of the daily value of vitamin B2.

4. Mushrooms

Mushrooms are not only a great source of selenium but also a great source of vitamin B2. Mushroom varieties, especially portabella, contain a good amount of vitamin B2. Even button mushrooms can meet your

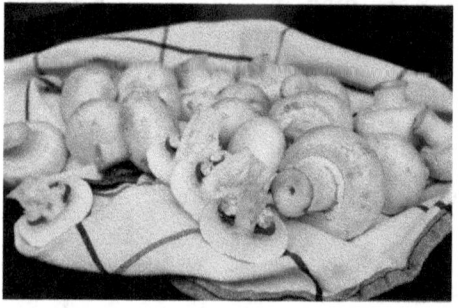

daily needs of vitamin B2. 1 cup of grilled portabella mushrooms can meet 30% of your daily requirement of vitamin B2, while 1 cup of button or white mushrooms can meet 22% of your daily requirement of vitamin B2.

5. Quinoa

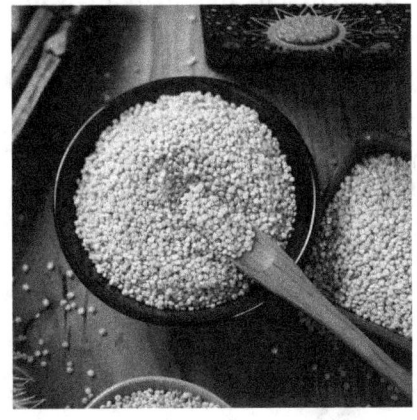

Quinoa is rich in quality protein, fiber, and many vitamins and minerals, including riboflavin. Quinoa is a complete protein, as it contains all essential nine amino acids your body needs. It is good for gut health, promotes digestion, reduces inflammation, and helps manage blood sugar levels. It keeps you energetic throughout the day and protects you from eye diseases. 1 cup of cooked quinoa meets 38% of the daily requirement of riboflavin.

6. Spinach

Spinach has an impressive nutrient profile. It has so many health benefits that it is considered a superfood. It is good for your eyesight.

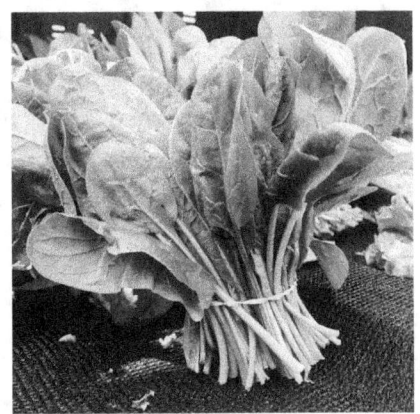

The high potassium content in it helps control high blood pressure. It is low in fat and high in water content, making it a weight loss friendly food. Spinach contains high amounts of antioxidants like zeaxanthin and carotenoids, these antioxidants kill free radicals in your body and prevent various types of cancer. 1 cup of cooked spinach fulfills 33% of the body's daily requirement of riboflavin.

7. Kidney Beans

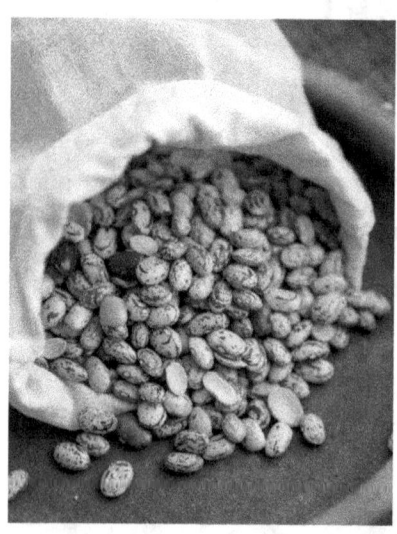

Kidney beans are not just named because of their kidney-like shape, they are actually good for your kidneys. They are high in magnesium and potassium, the deficiency of which can lead to kidney stones. They are high in soluble and insoluble fiber and low in fat, which promotes heart health and helps keep your blood pressure under control. They are an important source of vitamin B2. 1 cup of cooked red kidney beans meets 8% of the daily value of vitamin B2.

8. Soybeans

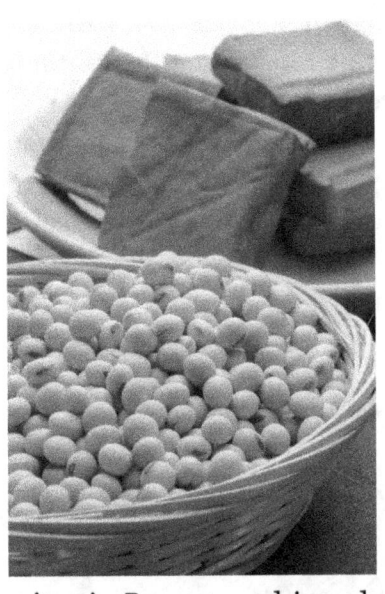

Soybeans are an excellent source of vitamin B2. They are also rich in heart-friendly fats like omega-3 and omega-6 and vitamin E. Soybeans have a good amount of protein and fiber that keep you feeling full for a long time. 1 cup of cooked soybeans contains 38% of the vitamin B2 you need in a day. Soybean is a versatile legume, you can dry roast them or make soy milk or tofu and use them in various recipes.

9. Apples

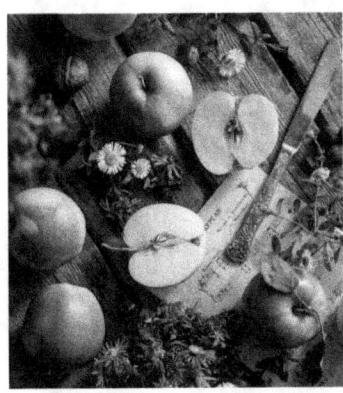

Apples are packed with a range of nutrients including fiber, vitamin B2, and vitamin C. They keep your digestion healthy and promote brain health. Digesting an apple burns more calories than eating an apple itself, making it a favorable snack for weight watchers. Do not forget to eat the apple with its peel. You may be surprised to know that apple peel contains more nutrition than the mass and eating apples with peel provides more nutrition than eating apples without peel. However, do not forget to wash the apples thoroughly to remove any amount of wax or pesticides from commercial farming practices. 1 large apple eaten with the peel can provide you with 8% daily value of vitamin B2.

10. Avocado

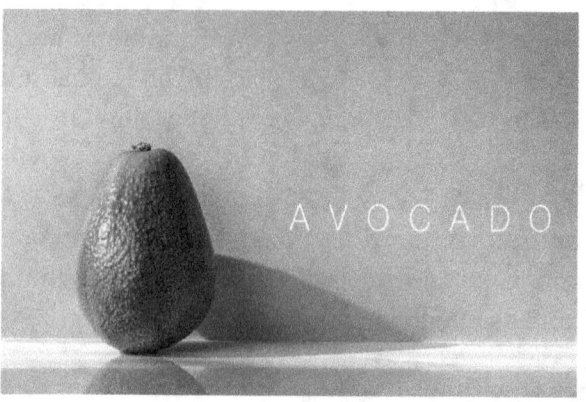

Avocados are rich in monounsaturated fats, but did you know they also provide a great range of water-soluble vitamins? They contain vitamins B2, B3, B5, B6 and folate. 1 medium-sized (136 g) avocado contains 15% of the daily requirement of vitamin B2. They are low in sodium and have no cholesterol. However, eat them in moderation because along with high monounsaturated fats, they also contain a good amount of saturated fats, which can be dangerous for your heart if eaten in large quantities.

Chapter 3
VITAMIN B3

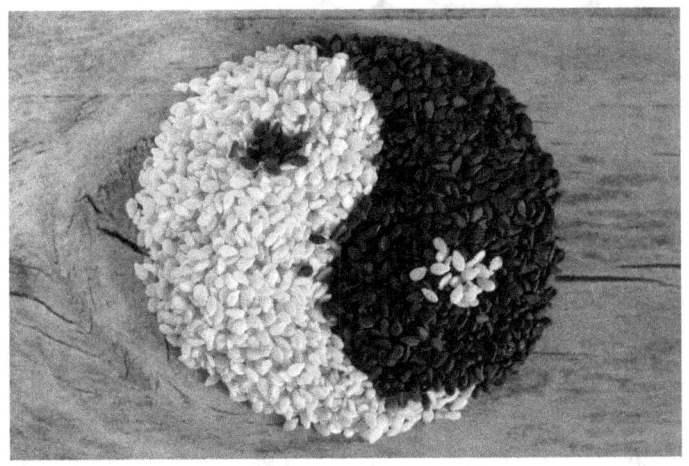

1.
EVERYTHING YOU NEED TO KNOW ABOUT VITAMIN B3

What is vitamin B3, and what does it do?

Niacin, a versatile nutrient also known as vitamin B3, is a water-soluble essential vitamin that your body needs daily through food. Niacin is also referred to nicotinic acid, nicotinamide and related derivatives, such as nicotinamide riboside and inositol hexanicotinate. Niacin is needed to convert carbohydrates, fats, and proteins into energy–adenosine triphosphate (ATP). It is also necessary for cellular communication, synthesis of cholesterol and fatty acids, and maintaining antioxidant function in your body.

What are the active forms of niacin?

Niacin is converted in your body into the metabolically active form, nicotinamide adenine dinucleotide (NAD), and acts as a coenzyme. NAD participates in more reactions in your body than any other coenzyme derived from vitamins. More than 400 enzymes require NAD to facilitate chemical reactions in your body. NAD can be converted to another active coenzyme form, called nicotinamide adenine dinucleotide phosphate (NADP), in all tissues except skeletal muscle. Niacin performs all of its biological activities through its active forms, NAD and NADP.

Tryptophan is an amino acid which is used in the synthesis of proteins. Tryptophan rich food are also considered a source of vitamin B3 because your body converts some of the tryptophan into NAD. However, this conversion only occurs when you consume enough protein. Therefore, the amount of niacin in your body is also influenced by your protein intake.

How is vitamin B3 metabolized in the body?

Most vitamin B3 or niacin in foods is in the form of nicotinic acid and nicotinamide, but the active forms NAD and NADP are also present in some foods that contain small amounts of NAD and NADP.

When you eat a niacin-rich diet, they are mostly absorbed in the small intestine; some residue is also absorbed in the stomach. However, when you consume food containing NAD and NADP, they are first converted to nicotinamide in the intestine and then absorbed.

When you take niacin supplements, after absorption, the required amount of niacin is metabolized to NAD. Excess niacin is taken up by the blood to form a reserve pool. Any remaining excess amount of niacin is converted to methylated forms by the liver, and then excreted through urine.

Are nicotinic acid and nicotinamide related to the nicotine found in tobacco?

No. Although they have similar names, neither nicotinic acid nor nicotinamide are related to the nicotine found in tobacco.

Is vitamin B3 stored in the body?

Like other water-soluble vitamins, vitamin B3 is stored poorly in your body. Niacin lasts a very short time in the body and is rapidly degraded, so you need a constant supply of it from the diet.

Is vitamin B3 really an essential nutrient?

An essential nutrient means that the nutrient cannot be made by the body and you must obtain it through food. Your liver can use tryptophan, an amino acid, to produce vitamin B3 or niacin. This conversion is only possible with a high-protein diet. Also, to convert tryptophan to niacin, your body must have adequate iron, vitamin B2, and vitamin B6 levels. Although your body can meet some of your daily needs by converting tryptophan into niacin, but it is an important vitamin that your body needs a constant supply of, so it's considered an essential nutrient that you must obtain through food every day.

How much vitamin B3 do I need a day?

The daily average recommended intake of niacin sufficient to meet the body's requirements for this nutrient is called the Recommended Dietary Allowance (RDA), and the range for almost all healthy individuals is given below:

Age	Male	Female
Birth to 6 m*	2 mg	2 mg
7–12 m*	4 mg NE	4 mg NE
1–3 yrs.	6 mg NE	6 mg NE
4–8 yrs.	8 mg NE	8 mg NE
9–13 yrs.	12 mg NE	12 mg NE
14+ yrs.	16 mg NE	14 mg NE

* Adequate Intake: Assumed level to ensure nutritional adequacy.

The RDA for niacin is expressed in milligrams of niacin equivalents (NE).

1 NE = 1 mg niacin = amino acid tryptophan. This means that the body converts 60 mg of the amino acid tryptophan into 1 mg niacin.

Adequate intake for infants from birth to 6 months indicates niacin alone since all the protein consumed by infants is used for development and growth.

What factors are responsible for niacin deficiency?

Poor diet: A diet lacking in vitamin B3 can lead to vitamin B3 deficiency. This can be due to a restricted diet or a diet lacking a variety of fruits and vegetables.

Inadequate intake of vitamin B2, vitamin B6 and iron

The enzymes needed to convert tryptophan to niacin require vitamins B2, B6, and iron to work. If you are deficient in vitamin B2, vitamin B6, and iron, you convert less tryptophan into niacin.

Certain disorders: Certain diseases such as inflammatory bowel disease, liver cirrhosis, anorexia, AIDS, and alcoholism can either reduce the absorption of niacin in your body or increase its excretion through urine or both, which can result in low niacin levels and even vitamin B3 deficiency.

Carcinoid syndrome: Carcinoid syndrome occurs when cancerous tumors called carcinoids in the gastrointestinal tract release serotonin and other substances that cause symptoms such as facial flushing and diarrhea. In people with carcinoid syndrome, tryptophan is not converted into niacin; instead, it is preferentially oxidized into serotonin. As a result, tryptophan is less available in the body to be converted into niacin.

Hartnup disease: A rare genetic disorder called Hartnup disease interferes with the intestinal, kidney, and cellular transport processes of several amino acids, including tryptophan. This disease affects the absorption of tryptophan in the small intestine as well as increases its excretion in the urine through the kidneys. As a result, tryptophan is less available in the body to be converted into niacin.

What are the symptoms and signs of vitamin B3 deficiency?

Vitamin B3 deficiency causes the 4Ds - diarrhea, dermatitis, dementia, and if left untreated, severe deficiency can lead to the fourth D, i.e., death. These 4Ds usually occur in this order.

So, common deficiency symptoms involve the digestive system, skin and nervous system and are as follow:

Digestive system-related symptoms:

- Bright red tongue
- Inflammation of the mouth
- Abdominal pain
- Vomiting
- Constipation
- Ultimately leads to diarrhea

Skin related symptoms:

- Thick and scaly skin
- Brown pigmented rash on skin exposed to sunlight

Brain-related symptoms:
- Headache
- Disorientation
- Memory loss
- Visual hallucinations
- Dementia

What happens if I am deficient in vitamin B3?

Severe niacin deficiency can cause pellagra. All the symptoms mentioned above are stages of pellagra development. Severe deficiency causes pigmented rashes on the part of the skin that is exposed to sunlight. The skin becomes rough and looks like a sunburn. Pellagra also causes the tongue to turn red and disturbs the digestive system, leading to vomiting and diarrhea. Neurological symptoms of pellagra include fatigue, depression, headache, paranoia, and hallucinations. If pellagra is not treated, it causes anorexia and can be life-threatening.

What happens if I take too much niacin?

Niacin is a water-soluble vitamin that is readily excreted through urine, so no adverse effects have been seen to date from excess niacin intake through food. However, high doses of both nicotinic acid and nicotinamide taken as supplements or medicine may cause adverse effects such as flushing, hypotension, impaired glucose tolerance, impaired vision, and heartburn.

How is vitamin B3 deficiency diagnosed?

The urinary excretion method is the most sensitive and reliable method to determine niacin status, as niacin levels in the blood are not a reliable indicator of niacin status. However, this test indicates only niacin status and not body stores of niacin, as no biochemical test is available so far that suggests total body stores of niacin. In the urinary excretion method, the amount of two methylated metabolites of niacin, N1-methyl-nicotinamide and N1-methyl-2-pyridone-5-carboxamide, are measured, which indicates niacin status in the body. The excretion rate ranges of these two metabolites for this method are given below:

More than 17.5 μmol/day: Adequate niacin level

5.8 to 17.5 μmol/day: Low niacin level

Less than 5.8 micromol/day: Niacin deficiency

When niacin status in the body is poor, NAD levels also decrease while NADP levels remain relatively stable. Another measure of niacin status is to check the ratio of NAD to NADP concentrations in whole blood.

A niacin number below 130 indicates niacin deficiency.

When the niacin index, i.e., the ratio of erythrocyte NAD to NADP concentrations, is below 1, it indicates that a person is at risk of niacin deficiency.

2. IMPORTANCE OF VITAMIN B3

FUNCTIONS OF NIACIN IN THE BODY

Vitamin B3 is involved in oxidation-reduction reactions (redox reactions) and non-redox reactions in the body. Redox reactions are essential for normal function, growth, and reproduction. Oxidation-reduction reactions are essential for energy production and vital to immune functions. Vitamin B3 is required by more than 400 enzymes to catalyze reactions in the body for normal living and survival. As a part of enzymatic reactions, vitamin B3 has the following important functions in the body:

Energy Production

Niacin is critically important for energy production in your body. It is required to convert the potential energy in carbohydrates, fats and proteins into the cell's primary energy currency i.e. adenosine triphosphate (ATP). All tissues in your body convert vitamin B3 into the coenzyme form nicotinamide adenine dinucleotide (NAD), which is its main metabolically active form.

Glucose is oxidized with NAD, acting as a carrier of two-electron equivalents and resulting in the production of ATP during mitochondrial oxidative phosphorylation.

Synthesis of Cholesterol and Triglycerides

NADH (H for hydrogen) is the reduced form of NAD. NADH plays an important role as a cofactor in synthesizing triglycerides, while NADPH, the reduced form of NADP, is essential in synthesizing cholesterol and fatty acids.

The most important step in cholesterol synthesis is the production of mevalonate from HMG-CoA by HMG-CoA reductase. The enzyme involved in this conversion needs NADPH as a cofactor. This step is important because cholesterol-lowering drugs and statins target this step to reduce the production of LDL in your body.

Synthesis of Bile Acids and Steroid Hormones

Bile acid synthesis requires the enzymatic conversion of cholesterol into primary bile acids. The enzymes involved in this conversion require NADPH as a cofactor to perform their action. Bile acids cannot be synthesized efficiently without sufficient NADPH in your body.

All steroid hormones, such as progesterone, testosterone, aldosterone, estradiol, and cortisol, are synthesized from cholesterol. The main functional class of enzymes involved in steroid synthesis are hydroxysteroid dehydrogenase (HSD) enzymes, which are dependent on both reduced (NADPH) and oxidized forms (NADP+) of NADP and require them as cofactors to exhibit their action. A deficiency in vitamin B3 in the body negatively affects the production of these steroid hormones.

Maintain Cellular Antioxidant Function

Vitamin B3 maintains the antioxidant function of your body. Over production of free radicals due to oxidative stress can damage lipids (cell membranes) and proteins, making you susceptible to diseases. Oxidative stress is the major cause of many chronic diseases like diabetes, cancer, arthritis, and others. Vitamin B3 is important in protecting against damage to lipids and proteins. It protects against oxidative damage caused by lipid peroxidation and protein oxidation. The inhibitory effect of vitamin B3 is more pronounced against protein oxidation than lipid peroxidation.

The glutathione-glutaredoxin (GRX) system and the thioredoxin (TRX) system are the major antioxidant systems in your body for defense against oxidative stress. The reduced form of NAD, i.e. NADPH, is part of both these antioxidant systems. NADPH acts as an essential cofactor in the reductive reactions involved in glutathione/lipid peroxidation. It inhibits the initial step of lipid peroxidation and thus prevents oxidation of lipids. NADPH is also involved in thioredoxin defense against oxidative stress. The thioredoxin antioxidant system reduces oxidative stress through disulfide reductase activity and regulates protein dithiol/disulfide balance. It plays an important role in immune oxidative defense responses.

Maintenance of Genome Integrity

NAD, the active niacin metabolite, is important in maintaining genome integrity, cell signaling, and DNA repair pathways. The status of the oxidized form of NAD in your body affects genomic stability. NAD participates in several ADP-ribosylation reactions that play important roles in maintaining genomic stability, gene expression, DNA repair, and cellular communication.

Aids in Calcium Signaling

Calcium signaling is a vital process in which calcium ions communicate and drive cellular activities in the body through their role as a second messenger. It is essentially involved in vital processes such as the secretion of insulin from beta cells in the pancreas, muscle cell contraction, the transfer of information between neurons in the brain, and T-lymphocyte activation in the immune system.

The classes of enzymes that catalyze the production of key calcium signaling regulators depend on the vitamin B3 coenzymes, NAD and NADP. These regulators work within cells to stimulate the release of calcium ions from storage sites such as mitochondria as well as to stimulate extracellular calcium entry through the cell membrane. Niacin deficiency in your body disrupts calcium signaling, making you prone to chronic diseases.

Natural Detoxification

NADP is necessary for the regeneration of detoxification components. The cells in your body expend a lot of energy to keep NADP in its reduced form, as it is used to reactivate oxidized compounds that can again participate in detoxification.

Your liver detoxifies harmful agents such as toxins, drugs, heavy metals, and preservatives. The detoxification process mainly involves the microsomal monooxygenase system. Cytochrome P-450 (CYP) are enzymes that are involved in converting insoluble organic compounds into water-soluble compounds, causing these to break down and release toxins or other harmful agents stored in the liver back into the bloodstream, which is then excreted through urine. Your body requires the constant availability of cytochrome P-450 (CYP) enzymes that can be regenerated for reuse by NADPH-dependent enzymes cytochrome P450 reductases (CPRs). Without enough niacin in your body, your liver cannot detoxify effectively.

TOP HEALTH BENEFITS OF VITAMIN B3

1. Prevent Cancer: Chronically inadequate levels of niacin in your body may increase the risk of cancer. Adequate vitamin B3 intake through dietary sources is associated with a reduced risk of several types of cancer, including breast, skin, oral, pharyngeal, esophageal, and lung cancer. NAD, the active form of vitamin B3, is essential for genome stability. Niacin deficiency reduces the amount of NAD in your body, which negatively affects NAD-dependent enzymes involved in maintaining genome stability and leads to damage to DNA and chromosomes, a hallmark of cancer. Low levels of NAD reduce the levels of tumor suppressor proteins. The enzymatic reactions responsible for DNA repair after DNA injury or DNA strand breaks depend on NAD concentration. Impaired DNA repair processes due to niacin deficiency may result in genome instability and lead to tumor development.

2. Improves Skin Health: Vitamin B3 deficiency can make your skin overly sensitive to sunlight. Niacin has a protective effect on the skin. It is involved in enhancing the skin barrier function and reducing the risk of ultraviolet rays-induced skin damage. Low levels of NAD increase oxidative stress, which causes DNA damage in the skin cells. Adequate vitamin B3 intake through diet enhances the response of skin cells to photodamage. Vitamin B3 acts as an antioxidant and prevents oxidative stress in the skin's lipid barrier, thus enhancing the integrity of the skin barrier and protecting against sun damage.

3. Lower Risk of Type-1 Diabetes Mellitus: Taking niacin through dietary sources is associated with a lower risk of type-1 diabetes. Sometimes, the immune system mistakenly attacks the beta cells in the pancreas that produce insulin, eventually destroying them and resulting in type 1 diabetes. Niacin has a protective effect on beta cells. It is involved in calcium signaling, which is necessary for insulin release from beta-cells. It acts as an anti-inflammatory and antioxidant agent. It reduces inflammation-related parameters as well as prevents oxidative damage to beta cells by neutralizing free radicals. However, this protective effect is only possible through dietary intake of niacin, not vitamin supplements. Studies have shown that high doses of nicotinic acid supplements can increase blood sugar levels by causing insulin resistance and increasing glucose production in the liver.

4. Lowering LDL Cholesterol and Cardioprotective Effects: Niacin plays an essential role in protection against cardiovascular diseases, it can improve your blood lipid profile and help slow the progression of atherosclerotic disease. Vitamin B3 in the form of nicotinic acid is used as a cholesterol-lowering drug. It improves the balance between bad (V) low-density lipoprotein (LDL) and good high-density lipoprotein (HDL). Niacin reduces VLDL and triglyceride levels and increases HDL level.

After lipids are broken down in adipose tissue, they are used to make VLDL in the liver, which eventually forms LDL. Nicotinic acid binds to a receptor in adipose tissue and inhibits fat breakdown. Since niacin inhibits fat breakdown, it decreases the free fatty acids in the circulation. This results in reduced hepatic triacylglycerol formation and increased apo B breakdown, which in turn inhibits very low-density lipoprotein (VLDL) secretion and impairs cholesterol biosynthesis.

High HDL levels are associated with reduced cardiovascular disease. The main protein component of HDL is apoA1, which prevents cardiovascular disease. Niacin increases HDL by reducing the breakdown of apoA1. Vitamin B3 selectively prevents the removal or uptake of HDL-apoA1 in your liver, thereby enhancing the ability of HDL-apoA1 to increase cholesterol efflux via the reverse cholesterol transport pathway.

5. Prevent and Treat Fatty Liver: Niacin may be effective in treating non-alcoholic fatty liver disease (NAFLD). Non-alcoholic fatty liver disease (NAFLD) refers to a condition in which a person's liver has too much fat that is not caused by excessive alcohol consumption. This condition is common worldwide, with one in 3 people having NAFLD. The active form of niacin, NAD, is an important target for preventing and treating fatty liver. It may improve fatty liver by reducing liver fat content, reducing liver inflammation, and preventing liver scarring.

6. May Improve Osteoarthritis Conditions:
High intake of vitamin B3 is associated with reduced pain and improved function in people with osteoarthritis. A form of vitamin B3, niacinamide may improve the overall condition of osteoarthritis and help reduce the amount of standard anti-inflammatory drugs NSAIDs (non-steroidal anti-inflammatory drugs) in treatment. It improves joint flexibility and reduces inflammation by inhibiting inflammation-causing agents in your body, thereby reducing swelling and persistent pain associated with osteoporosis.

7. Prevent Age-Related Cognitive Decline:
Vitamin B3, especially the nicotinamide form, is important for developing and maintaining the central nervous system. Low levels of vitamin B3 can lead to slow mental processes, brain fog, and cognitive decline. Vitamin B3 protects brain cells through various mechanisms. It is a key mediator of the growth and survival of brain cells. It increases the production of nitric oxide (NO), a vasodilator that relaxes and dilates the blood vessels in your brain; this increases oxygen and nutrient-rich blood flow to your brain. Niacin gives your brain a constant and sustained energy supply due to its role in ATP production. It acts as an antioxidant and helps eliminate free radicals that can damage nerve cells. It improves cognitive function by

stimulating the production of dopamine neurotransmitters, which enhance mood, memory, learning, and cognitive performance. High dietary niacin intake helps protect against stroke, Alzheimer's, Parkinson's, dementia, and mental disorders.

8. Prevent Cataracts: High intake of vitamin B3 through diet is associated with a reduced risk of developing cataracts. Oxidative damage to lens proteins due to oxidative stress is a major cause of the initiation and development of cataract formation, the most common cause of blindness in the world today. Vitamin B3 derivative, NAD, improves and protects nerve cell function and prevents damage to the optic nerve. Vitamin B3 from fruits and vegetables has a protective effect on the eyes and does not have any side effects. However, vitamin B3 supplements should be taken cautiously and only under medical supervision as high doses of niacin have adverse effects on the eyes, causing blurred vision, inflammation of the cornea, and macular damage.

3.
10 RICHEST VEGETARIAN SOURCES OF VITAMIN B3

In vegetarian food sources, niacin is mainly present as nicotinic acid. In some grains, niacin is available in the bond of polysaccharides and glycopeptides. Due to this bond, the bioavailability of niacin is reduced by 30%. Tryptophan, one of the essential amino acids, is also considered a good source of niacin. Tryptophan is converted to niacin when it is present in the body in adequate amounts, i.e., more than the amount required for protein synthesis. It is mainly converted to the active form of niacin, i.e., NAD in the liver. The standard ratio in which tryptophan is converted to NAD is 1:60, i.e., 60 mg of tryptophan produces 1 mg of niacin (NAD).

Below are the top 10 vegetarian food sources of Vitamin B3 (Niacin):

1. Brown Rice and Whole Wheat

Brown rice is a rich source of vitamin B3. Niacin, or vitamin B3, is present in the outer fibrous layer called bran. In brown rice, only the inedible part, the hull, is removed while the bran, germ, and endosperm layers are left intact, whereas in white rice, the processing removes the outer two nutritious bran and germ layers, and only the carbohydrate-rich endosperm left, leaving very few essential nutrients. Due to the hard bran layer, brown rice takes more time to cook compare to white rice, which cooks quickly. Similarly, processing of refined flour removes the bran layer and does not leave much vitamin B3, while whole wheat has a good amount of vitamin B3 due to the bran layer. 1 cup of cooked brown rice can fulfill 33% of your daily requirement of vitamin B3, and 100 g of whole wheat flour contains 33% of your body's daily requirement of vitamin B3.

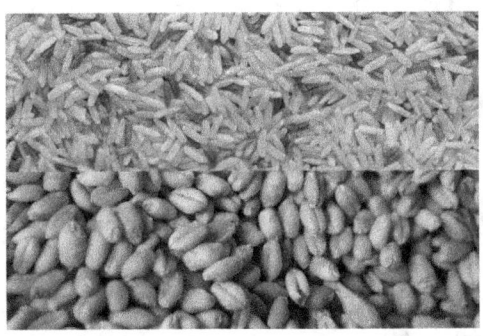

2. Peanuts

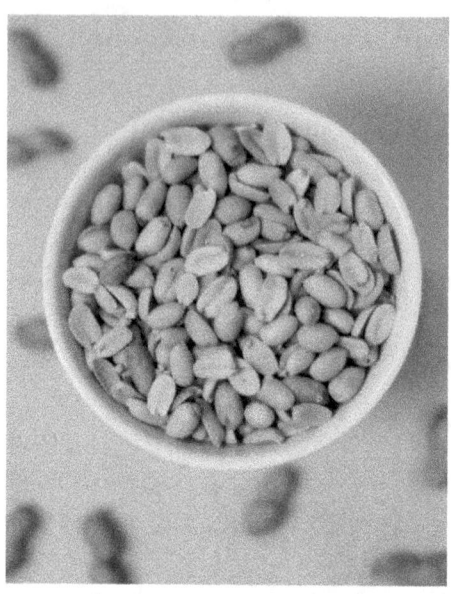

Peanuts are one of the best sources of vitamin B3. Not just vitamin B3, it contains a good amount of protein, magnesium, manganese, phosphorus, and vitamin B6 and is loaded with monounsaturated and polyunsaturated fats, which are heart-friendly fats. Although peanuts contain more good fats than saturated fats and do not cause weight gain but eat them in moderation as they are high in omega-6 fats. Omega-6 fats can increase inflammation in the body when consumed in abundance and not in balance with omega-3 fats. Inflammation can lead to chronic diseases like rheumatoid arthritis and diabetes and increase your cholesterol levels, which ultimately affects heart health. A handful of dry roasted peanuts fulfills 26% daily value of vitamin B3.

3. Potatoes and Sweet

Potatoes and sweet potatoes are both good sources of vitamin B3. Peeling or not peeling potatoes and sweet

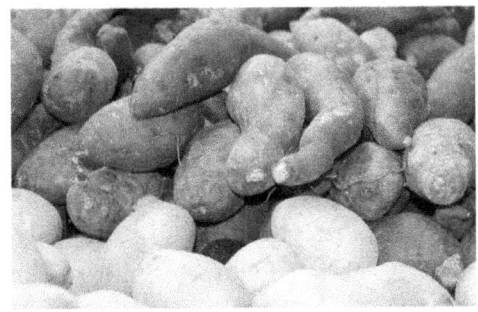

potatoes does not affect their niacin content. 1 large baked sweet potato (180 grams) can meet 17% of the daily requirement of niacin and 1 medium-large baked potato (180 grams) can meet 16% of your body's daily niacin requirement. Including potatoes and sweet potatoes in your diet can be a good way to increase your niacin consumption.

4. Sunflower Seeds

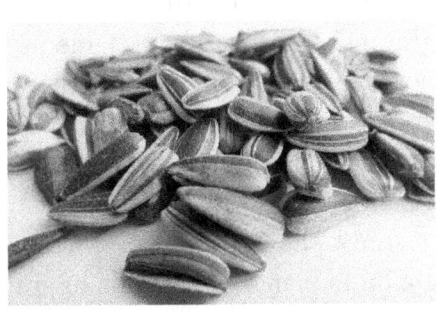

Sunflower seeds are rich in healthy fatty acids, protein, and free radical-killing antioxidants that help reduce the risk of developing chronic diseases. A handful of dry-roasted sunflower seeds can provide 13% of your daily recommended dose of vitamin B3. They are healthy snacks that keep you energized throughout the day by ensuring a constant energy supply to your organs. They help lower your blood pressure naturally through their magnesium and linoleic acid content, both of which are excellent in promoting low blood pressure and ultimately protect you from cardiovascular diseases.

5. Seeds

Sesame seeds are a great source of tryptophan, an amino acid that converts into vitamin B3 in the body. Tryptophan is also essential for the synthesis of serotonin and melatonin, the sleep-regulating hormones. Sesame seeds help you sleep better, keep you in a happy mood, and are great for your hair health. A handful (28 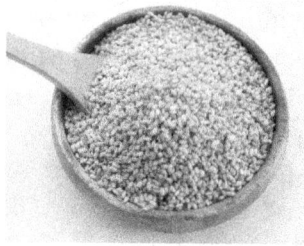 grams) of dry roasted sesame seeds can fulfill 8% of your daily vitamin B3 requirement. Black sesame seeds are considered slightly better than white sesame seeds as they are more nutritious and contain more iron, calcium, potassium, copper, and manganese. However, a study showed that sprouted white sesame seeds contained more tryptophan than sprouted black sesame seeds.

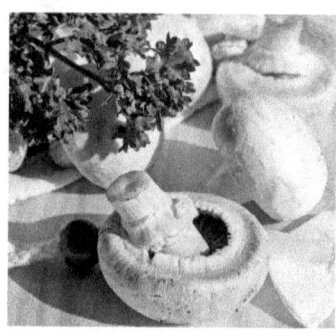

6. Button Mushrooms

Mushrooms are a good source for vegetarians to get more niacin. Mushrooms are rich in selenium, vitamin D (if you are buying UV-exposed mushrooms), and vitamin B6, along with vitamin B3. It supports a healthy immune system, weight loss, and bone health and helps lower your cholesterol levels. It does wonders for your hair due to its high selenium content. 100 g of button mushrooms contain 24% of your daily requirement of vitamin B3.

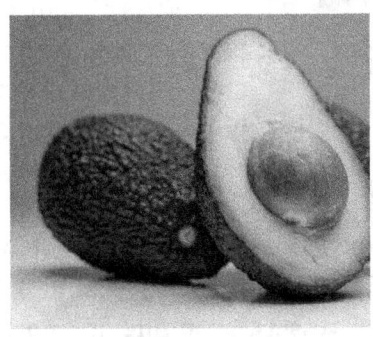

7. Avocados

Avocados are a versatile fruit. They are popular for their high monounsaturated fat content, but their health-benefiting properties are not just limited to their healthy fats. They contain a wide range of nutrients and are rich in water-soluble and fat-soluble vitamins such as vitamins C, B2, B3, B5, B6, B9, and vitamins E and K. You may be surprised to know that avocados contain more than twice the potassium than bananas and are a great fruit for managing your blood pressure. One medium-sized avocado (136 grams) contains 16% of the RDA of niacin. However, like any other high-fat food, overconsumption of avocados can lead to weight gain and body fat storage, so consume them in moderation.

8. Mango

Mango is an excellent source of fiber and vitamin C. It is high in vitamin A, folate, and vitamin B3. One mango

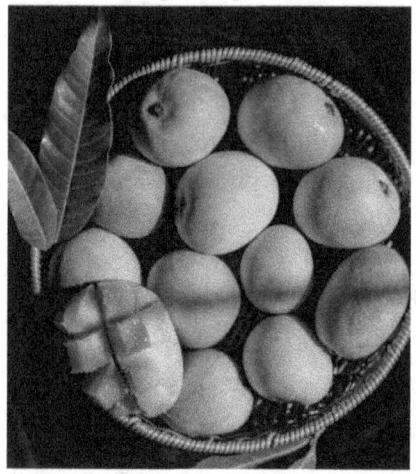

(about 325g-350g) can fulfill 15% of your daily requirement of niacin. It is good for digestion and reduces constipation. The antioxidant properties of mango promote eye health and strengthen your immune system. Vitamin C in mango increases iron absorption in your body, increasing hemoglobin formation and RBC production. Moreover, vitamin B3 helps widen your blood vessels, resulting in more oxygen and nutrient-rich blood reaching your organs seamlessly, keeping them healthy and working efficiently.

9. Lentils

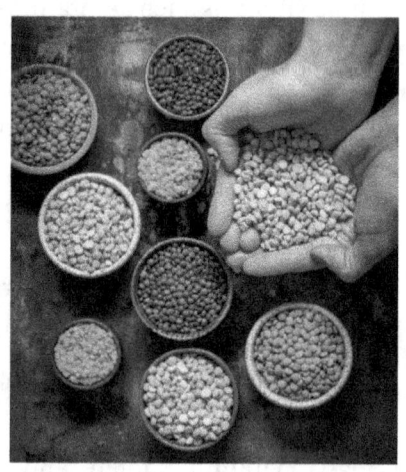

Lentils like split pigeon peas, split mung beans, split red lentils, and split Bengal gram are excellent sources of vitamin B3. They are also rich in protein, fiber, other B vitamins, and minerals such as iron, zinc, potassium, and magnesium. They help you prevent anemia and chronic diseases such as diabetes, obesity, and cardiovascular diseases. They are low glycemic index foods, so they prevent sudden spikes of glucose in your blood and help manage blood sugar levels. One cup of cooked lentils contains 12% of the daily value of vitamin B3.

10. Green Peas

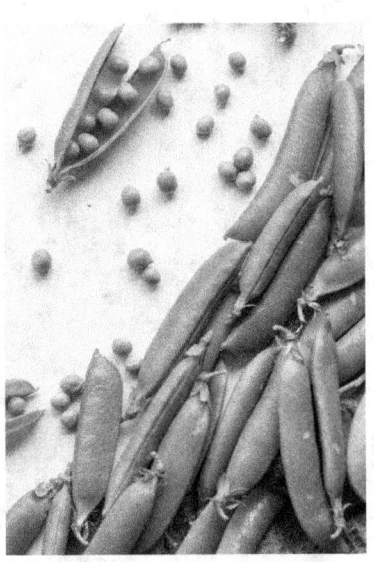

Green peas are a good source of vitamin B3. 1 cup of cooked green peas provides 20% of your daily recommended intake of niacin. They are fibrous and high-protein vegetarian sources. Their high fiber content makes them a gut-friendly vegetable or, more precisely, a gut-friendly legume. Antioxidants like vitamins C and E in green peas strengthen your immune system and protect you from infections. The anti-inflammatory agents present in green peas reduce inflammation, which reduces your risk of developing chronic disorders like diabetes, arthritis, cancer, and cardiovascular diseases.

Chapter 4
VITAMIN B5

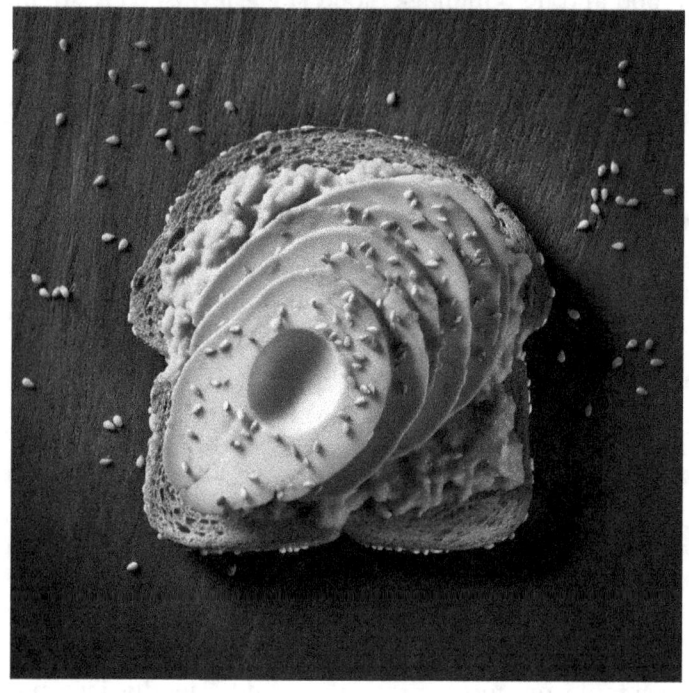

1.
EVERYTHING YOU NEED TO KNOW ABOUT VITAMIN B5

What is Vitamin B5, and what does it do?

Vitamin B5 is an essential water-soluble vitamin, also known as pantothenic acid. Its primary function is in the synthesis of coenzyme A (CoA) and acyl carrier proteins, which are essential for fatty acid synthesis and other metabolic processes in the body.

How does vitamin B5 metabolize in the body?

About 85% of food contains pantothenic acid. It is usually present as a component of coenzyme A or phosphopantetheine. When you consume these foods, the digestive enzymes in your intestinal lumen and intestinal cells convert these forms into pantothenic acid. Pantothenic acid is then absorbed in your intestine, taken up by red blood cells, and circulated throughout your body. The dephosphorylated form of phosphopantetheine, i.e., pantetheine, is first converted into pantothenic acid by intestinal cells and then transported into your bloodstream.

Is vitamin B5 stored in the body?

Vitamin B5 is a water-soluble vitamin, so it does not stay in your body for long, nor does your body store it for later use. Your body only absorbs the amount needed to perform bodily functions. Any excess vitamin B5 you take is excreted through urine without being stored for later use. This means that you need to get vitamin B5 from dietary sources daily to maintain optimal levels of vitamin B5 in your body.

Is vitamin B5 really an essential nutrient?

Yes, vitamin B5 is an essential nutrient that you must get from dietary sources daily to maintain healthy levels of vitamin B5 in your body. Your intestinal flora may also produce some pantothenic acid, but how much of it your body absorbs isn't yet known. So until we have more information on this, vitamin B5 is considered an essential nutrient.

How much vitamin B5 do I need a day?

The Recommended Dietary Allowance (RDA) is established when enough information is available to determine the required amount of a nutrient per day for approximately 97% to 98% of healthy individuals. If not, the Estimated Average Requirement (EAR) is established, which indicates the amount of a nutrient required by 50% of healthy individuals to meet the body's requirements. As the data for pantothenic acid is insufficient to obtain the EAR, the Adequate Intake (AI) for vitamin B5 or pantothenic acid is established. It indicates the level of vitamin B5 intake to ensure nutritional adequacy. Below are the Adequate Intakes (AI) for pantothenic acid.

Age	Male	Female
Birth to 6 m	1.7 mg	1.7 mg
7–12 m	1.8 mg	1.8 mg
1–3 yrs.	2 mg	2 mg
4–8 yrs.	3 mg	3 mg
9–13 yrs.	4 mg	4 mg
14+ yrs.	5 mg	5 mg

What are the factors that can lead for pantothenic acid deficiency?

Vitamin B5 deficiency is very rare as it is found in almost all foods. However, certain factors can lead to vitamin B5 deficiency:

Severe malnourishment: Only case of severe malnourishment in specific cases when a person gets very limited food may develop vitamin B5 deficiency. The deficiency can be relieved by pantothenic acid supplementation.

Certain drugs: Vitamin B5 deficiency can occur un people who are consuming pantothenic acid antagonist such as omega-methylpantothenic acid.

Pantothenate kinase-associated neurodegeneration 2 mutation: Pantothenic acid kinase is an enzyme that is needed for CoA and phosphopantetheine production. Mutations in the pantothenate kinase 2 (PANK2) gene cause a rare, inherited disorder called pantothenate kinase-associated neurodegeneration (PKAN) which is associated with brain iron accumulation. A large number of PANK2 mutations reduce the activity of pantothenate kinase 2 which potentially decrease the conversion of pantothenic acid to CoA and thus loewring CoA levels.

What are the signs and symptoms of vitamin B5 deficiency?

While pantothenic acid Deficiency is not common but those who are deficient in pantothenic acid have following signs:

- Weakness
- Headache
- Insomnia
- Depression
- Disturbed Sleep,
- Irritability

- Restlessness
- Numbness and tingling of the hands and feet
- Gastrointestinal distress with anorexia

What happens if I have insufficient levels of vitamin B5 in my body?

Fatigue: Vitamin B5 takes part in converting food into energy which is used by each cell to perform its functions. Deficiency of vitamin B5 affects ATP production. Since your body is unable to effectively convert glucose into energy (ATP), resulting in fatigue and weakness.

Hyperlipidemia: Pantothenic acid has a vital role in triglyceride synthesis and lipoprotein metabolism. It helps control triglyceride and cholesterol levels in your body. When you have low levels of vitamin B5 your body, it fails to reduce lipid levels and may result in hyperlipidemia.

Hair loss: Vitamin B5 boosts the growth of hair cells. Vitamin B5 deficiency causes the hair follicles to become malnourished, leading to reduced hair growth and, eventually, hair loss.

Graying of hair: Vitamin B5 potentially slows down the process of graying of hair. It promotes the growth of hair cells. Inadequate levels of vitamin B5 in your body accelerate the process of graying of hair, which can be reversed by increasing your dietary vitamin B5 intake.

Alzheimer's disease: People with Alzheimer's disease are often found to be deficient in vitamin B5. Vitamin B5 is essential for energy production (ATP) and helps keep the brain active. Vitamin B5 deficiency may lead to neurodegenerative Alzheimer's disease.

Huntington's disease: Vitamin B5 deficiency can lead to age-related dementia-like Huntington's disease. Acetylcholine is a neurotransmitter that facilitates proper nerve signaling. Vitamin B5 plays an essential role in the synthesis of acetylcholine. A deficiency in vitamin B5 cause deficiency of acetylcholine whch causes degeneration of neurons and loss of myelin leading to Huntington's disease.

Poor wound healing: Pantothenic acid speeds up the normal healing process. It improves wound healing, especially after surgery. It moisturizes the skin and enhances the skin's barrier function. Low levels of vitamin B5 negatively affect the wound healing process. Its deficiency also reduces immunity power, which is essential for wound healing. As a result, your wound does not heal quickly.

Poor skin health: Vitamin B5 is often added to skin products as it moisturizes the skin, prevents skin reactions, and keeps it healthy. Inadequate levels of vitamin B5 make the skin vulnerable to infections and affect overall skin health.

Poor immune response: Vitamin B5 regulates the innate immune response by regulating CoA levels. Vitamin B5 has a pro-inflammatory effect on macrophages and helps fight infections. Inadequate levels of vitamin B5 in the body affect the immune response against infections and reduce your immunity power in fighting pathogens.

Does cooking affect the amount of vitamin B5 in food?

Yes, vitamin B5 is a heat-sensitive vitamin, which means it degrades at high temperatures. So, cooking food containing vitamin B5 reduces its vitamin B5 content by up to 67%.

What happens if I take too much pantothenic acid?

Pantothenic acid is readily excreted in the urine and does not store well in your body, so pantothenic acid does not cause toxicity in humans, even at high intakes. Taking vitamin B5 through dietary sources does not lead to very high levels in the body, however, this is not the case with pantothenic acid supplements. A 10 g/day dose of pantothenic acid causes mild diarrhea and gastrointestinal discomfort.

How is vitamin B5 deficiency diagnosed?

Vitamin B5 status is not typically measured in healthy people. However, the two methods below are primarily used to measure vitamin B5 status when necessary.

Urine Concentration

This is the primary method to determine pantothenic acid status in the body. It is the most reliable indicator of pantothenic acid status because of its close relationship with dietary intake.

The urinary excretion rate ranges for pantothenic acid are as follows:

About 2.6 mg of pantothenic acid per day: Normal

Less than 1 mg of pantothenic acid per day: Deficiency

Whole Blood Concentration

The whole blood concentration of pantothenic acid reflects your intake of pantothenic acid through diet. In this method, whole blood is first treated with enzymes to release free pantothenic acid from CoA and then the concentration of pantothenic acid is measured.

The blood concentration range of pantothenic acid is as follows:

1.6 to 2.7 mcmol/L: Normal

Less than 1 mcmol/L: Vitamin B5 deficiency

2. IMPORTANCE OF VITAMIN B5

The main function of vitamin B5 is to synthesize coenzyme-A (CoA) and acyl carrier proteins. All the vital functions in the body take place through coenzyme-A and acyl carrier proteins. There are two types of reactions in the body- catabolic and anabolic reactions. The catabolic process involves breaking down molecules and releasing energy, which is used by the body. In contrast, anabolic reactions involve the use of energy to form molecules, which are used by the body to function. An example of catabolism involves breaking down carbohydrates into energy, while an example of anabolism involves the synthesis of fatty acids in the body. The metabolically active components of vitamin B5, coenzyme-A, and acyl carrier proteins are involved in both catabolic and anabolic reactions. Some of the main functions of pantothenic acid are given below.

FUNCTIONS OF PANTOTHENIC ACID IN THE BODY

Production of Red Blood Cells

Pantothenic acid increases the production of red blood cells. Hemoglobin is an important part of red blood cells (RBCs) that gives them their red color and enables them to carry oxygen and deliver it to tissues and organs. RBCs deliver nutrients to tissues and organs that help them function normally. An active metabolite of pantothenic acid, coenzyme A is involved in the synthesis of porphyrin (heme), a component of hemoglobin. Without enough coenzyme A, your body cannot produce hemoglobin efficiently, resulting in low production of red blood cells. Therefore, vitamin B5 is needed for proper red blood cell production and normal body functioning.

Energy Production

Pantothenic acid is essentially required for energy metabolism. It serves as a cofactor in the synthesis of coenzyme A. Your body needs the active metabolite of pantothenic acid, coenzyme A, and its acyl derivatives to produce energy from the breakdown of fats, carbohydrates, and proteins from your food. Coenzyme A is important for the metabolism of fatty acids and the citric acid cycle for energy production.

Synthesis of Essential Fats and Cholesterol

Lipids are essential for normal body function. Vitamin B5 is involved in the biosynthesis of essential lipids such as phospholipids, sphingolipids, cholesterol, and bile salts. Fatty acid synthase (FAS) is a multienzyme complex system that induces the synthesis of fatty acids. Within the fatty acid synthase complex system, acyl-carrier protein (ACP) requires pantothenic acid as a prosthetic group for its activity as a carrier protein. Pantothenic acid derivatives such as acetyl-coenzyme A, malonyl-coenzyme A, and acyl-carrier protein are all essential for the synthesis of fatty acids. The acetyl-CoA form of vitamin B5 is required for cholesterol synthesis. Without adequate vitamin B5, your body cannot manufacture cholesterol, steroids, and other physiologically important lipids.

Hormone Production

Vitamin B5 can improve fertility rates, reduce stress, and help you sleep better at night. Vitamin B5 in the form of coenzyme A and its derivatives is important for producing various hormones in your body. It enables the synthesis of the stress hormone cortisol in the adrenal glands (small gland located on top of your kidney). In stressful situations, it increases the secretion of cortisol, and when the stress period is over, it reduces cortisol secretion and thus relieves anxiety. Coenzyme A derivatives are required for the synthesis of the melatonin hormone. Melatonin helps synchronize sleep-wake cycles and maintain the body's circadian rhythm (internal clock). In addition, pantothenic acid active compounds are involved in the synthesis of sex hormones and help in the early development of the fetus. Consuming foods rich in vitamin B5 in adequate amounts helps boost your reproductive health.

Neurotransmitters and Myelin Biosynthesis

Consistent energy, healthy nerve cells, and myelin sheath are the keys to keeping your brain at its best and protecting against neurodegenerative diseases such as dementia, Alzheimer's, and Huntington's. Pantothenic acid, as part of acetyl-coenzyme-A, is engaged in myelin biosynthesis. The myelin sheath is a protective layer that coats the main body part of nerve cells. The myelin sheath facilitates the quick transmission of electrical impulses along nerve cells. Acetylcholine is a neurotransmitter that facilitates proper nerve signaling and has a critical role in maintaining myelinated neurons. Vitamin B5-derived CoA is essential for synthesizing acetylcholine, which is responsible for various brain functions, including memory, heart contraction, blood pressure, and muscle control.

Detoxification

Your body has its own detoxification mechanism. Your liver detoxifies toxins by changing their chemical nature. Liver cells can convert toxic products, drugs such as sulfonamides, and alcohol into harmless byproducts, which can pass out of your system through urine. Pantothenic acid is involved in the detoxification process in the form of coenzyme A. Vitamin B5 is involved in beta-oxidation, the process of breaking down fatty acid molecules. The reactions in the liver that convert toxins into harmless products require coenzyme A. Without enough vitamin B5, your liver cannot perform this process and is unable to remove toxins from the body, which then accumulate and cause adverse effects.

Gene Expression

Vitamin B5 is essential for the genome and gene expression. Vitamin B5 is required for the biosynthesis of coenzyme A. All sequenced genomes encode enzymes that require coenzyme A as a substrate. Coenzyme A is involved in many acetylation reactions. It gets its name because of its role in acetylation reactions. Most acetylated proteins in your body are modified by acetyl-CoA (a form of coenzyme A) donating an acetate group. Histones, a type of protein that provides structural support for chromosomes, are acetylated by acetyl-CoA, which facilitates transcription (mRNA synthesis) and regulates gene expression.

TOP HEALTH BENEFITS OF VITAMIN B5

1. Reduce Cholesterol Levels in People with Dyslipidemia/Hyperlipidemia: Abnormal levels of lipids in the blood are called dyslipidemia, possibly due to lifestyle or genetic factors. An abnormal lipid profile can significantly increase your risk for cardiovascular diseases (CVD). Hyperlipidemia refers to increased levels of cholesterol and triglycerides in your blood. Since vitamin B5 is involved in triglyceride synthesis and the metabolism of lipids, pantethine, a form of pantothenic acid, can efficiently reduce lipid levels in people with hyperlipidemia and dyslipidemia. Pantothenic acid is important for the biosynthesis of coenzyme A, which is involved in the transport of fatty acids into cells and mitochondria. Pantethine has significant lipid-lowering potential, reducing low-density lipoprotein cholesterol (LDL) and triglyceride levels and increasing high-density lipoprotein cholesterol levels by inhibiting cholesterol synthesis and accelerating fatty acid breakdown in the mitochondria.

2. Promote Hair Health and Prevent Gray Hair: Vitamin B5 is a wonderful vitamin for your hair. Many hair products contain vitamin B5 because it has so many benefits. Vitamin B5 is a humectant that moisturizes and conditions the hair, giving your hair a shine and luster. It helps clear dead cells in the scalp and make room for new hair follicles to grow. It forms a protective layer around the hair shaft and protects it from damage caused by chemicals like coloring, shampooing, and mechanical processes like brushing and combing. It reduces the formation of split ends, improves manageability, and strengthens your hair.

High dietary intake of vitamin B5 or using shampoos containing pantothenic acid may prevent gray hair formation or even restore hair color. Recent research has shown promising effects of vitamin B5 in treating alopecia or male/female pattern hair loss. However, more research is needed to confirm and establish this finding.

3. Wound Healing: Pantothenic acid is important for the growth and maintenance of your skin health. Intake of vitamin B5 through food and applying it topically accelerates the wound healing process, especially after surgery. It has a moisturizing effect on the skin and enhances the skin's barrier function. It increases cellular multiplication and protein synthesis during the early postoperative period, which aids in tissue repair and, therefore, accelerates the wound healing process.

4. Better Skin Health: Vitamin B5 boosts your skin health. It is a common ingredient in various skin care products. Two forms of vitamin B5, dexpanthenol and panthenol, have been approved by the Food and Drug Administration (FDA) for use in skin care products. Vitamin B5 provides hydration, moisturizing, and emollient effects on the skin. It acts as a humectant and hydrates the top layer of your skin by attracting water from the lower layers of the skin and retaining moisture. Due to its emollient effect, it heals dry patches and prevents dryness, making your skin smooth and soft. Vitamin B5 strengthens your skin barrier, reduces moisture loss, and protects against environmental damage.

5. Prevent and Treat Mouth Ulcers: Eating a diet rich in vitamin B5 helps prevent mouth ulcers. It is effective in treating mouth ulcers. When taken with other B vitamins, vitamin B5 can accelerate the healing process of ulcers and reduce the time needed for treatment. It also greatly reduces the chances of mouth ulcers recurring.

6. Reduce Anxiety Levels: Vitamin B5 can help manage your stress. It can reduce anxiety and stress by regulating cortisol levels in the body. Vitamin B5 is essential for stress hormone production in the adrenal glands. Stress induces the production of cortisol, the stress hormone. When the stress signal is over, cortisol levels return to normal. However, chronic stress releases too much cortisol, which harms your body. Eating enough vitamin B5-rich foods helps your adrenal glands produce cortisol and ensures they don't produce too much or too little cortisol so your body can recover.

7. Boost Eye Health: Vitamin B5 boosts your eye health. It prevents dry eyes and other eye problems.

Vitamin B5 has moisturizing effects and promotes wound healing. It also has anti-inflammatory effects. Because of its moisturizing and anti-inflammatory properties, it helps keep your eyes lubricated, prevent eye inflammation, and speed up wound healing. In fact, dexpanthenol, a form of vitamin B5, is often used in eye drops to treat dry eyes as well as reduce pain and inflammation.

8. Prevent Age-Related Dementia: One of the most common reasons for age-related neurodegeneration and dementia is Alzheimer's disease (AD). Vitamin B5 deficiency plays a key role in Alzheimer's disease. A deficiency in this vitamin particularly affects the areas of the brain that are known to be severely damaged in AD. Your brain requires 20% of the total energy in the body. Vitamin B5 is converted into acetyl-CoA in the body, which plays a key role in making energy from food and producing ATP. This way it keeps your brain active and functional. Taking enough vitamin B5 can prevent and treat dementia caused by Alzheimer's disease.

3.
10 RICHEST VEGETARIAN SOURCES OF VITAMIN B5

Almost all edible foods contain pantothenic acid, but in varying amounts. Edible plant tissues contain high concentrations of pantothenic acid. However, these foods undergo food processing before they reach your table during which about 20% to 80% of these pantothenic acid dense plant tissues are destroyed. The absorption rate of pantothenic acid in the body is optimal. The body absorbs 40% to 60% of pantothenic acid from foods.

Some of the richest vegetarian sources of Vitamin B5 (pantothenic acid) are as follows:

1. Shiitake Mushrooms

Mushrooms are an excellent source of vitamin B5. 1 cup of grilled shiitake mushrooms fulfills more than 100% (about 104%) of your daily required vitamin B5. Button or white mushrooms also contain vitamin B5. 1 cup of cooked white mushrooms contains 32% of the daily requirement of vitamin B5. Shiitake mushrooms are so nutritious; in fact, their extract is also used for medicinal purposes. They effectively boost immune function, keep skin healthy and reduce bad cholesterol levels. But these mushrooms should be consumed with caution by people with autoimmune conditions such as rheumatoid arthritis as it can make your immune system more active and interfere with the way your anti-rheumatic medicines work.

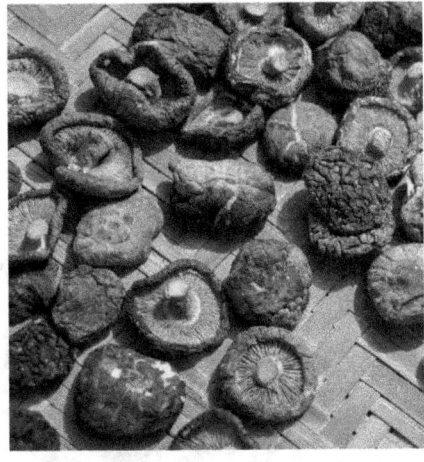

2. Sunflower Seeds

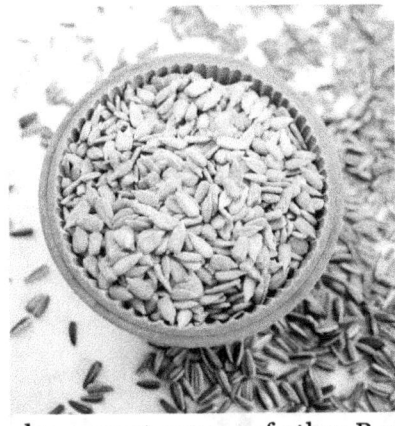

Sunflower seeds are an excellent source of vitamin B5. A quarter cup of sunflower seeds can fulfill almost 50% of your daily requirement of vitamin B5. They are also a great source of other B vitamins and fat-soluble vitamin E. Sunflower seeds are rich in healthy fats that keep your lipid profile normal and protect your heart from dysfunction. However, due to its high omega-6 fat content, people with inflammatory diseases like arthritis and IBS should consume these seeds in moderation as they can worsen your existing condition.

3. Avocado

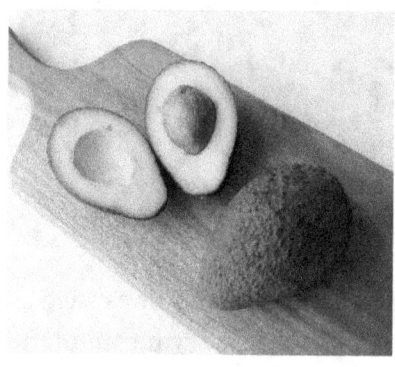

Consuming avocado in moderation can greatly increase vitamin B5 and monounsaturated fatty acids in your body. One raw avocado can meet 40% of your daily requirement of vitamin B5. The high vitamin content in avocado helps maintain healthy cellular function and keep you active. The high good monounsaturated fat content reduces inflammation in your body and prevents inflammatory diseases like osteoporosis.

4. Milk and Milk products

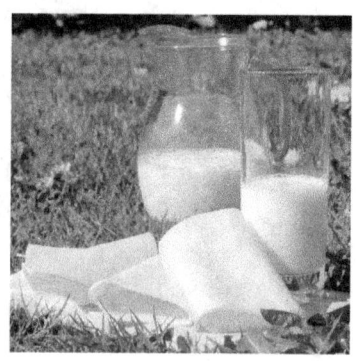

Milk and milk products are great sources to add vitamin B5 to your diet. One cup of 2% fat milk contains 18% of the daily requirement of vitamin

B5, while 1 cup of plain yogurt can fulfill 12% of daily recommended intake of vitamin B5. Milk and milk products are excellent sources of vitamins and minerals. The complete protein in milk can strengthen your body and help repair muscles after a workout.

5. Potatoes

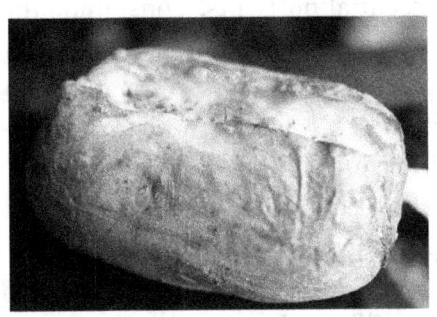

Potatoes have a bad reputation for being a starchy vegetable, but they can certainly fulfill some of your body's nutrient needs when it comes to vitamins and minerals. A baked potato with the skin can fulfill 14% of the daily value of vitamin B5. Include boiled potatoes in your diet instead of fried potatoes, and eat them with the skin because potato skins contain 12 times more antioxidants than pulp. Eating potatoes with the skin increases your total fiber intake compared to eating potatoes without the skin.

6. Peanuts

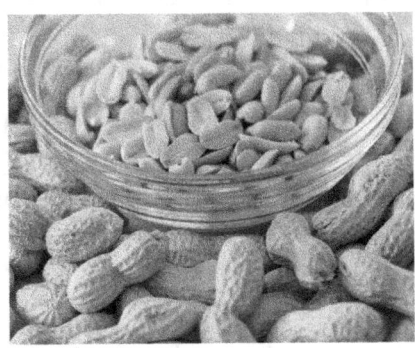

Peanuts are a good source of vitamin B5. Half a cup of peanuts roasted in oil fulfills 20% of the daily vitamin B5 requirement of your body. They are rich in protein, good fats, fiber and lots of essential vitamins and minerals. They contain more protein than any other nuts, which makes you feel full for a long time and aids in weight loss. A handful of peanuts is enough to provide your body with the essential nutrients. Consuming them in excess can do more harm than good. Excessive consumption of peanuts increases inflammation and makes you vulnerable to inflammatory diseases. Also, they can interfere with the absorption of iron, zinc, and calcium. They can make you gain weight and impair your digestion. So, eat them in moderation.

7. Broccoli

Broccoli is rich in vitamin B5. 1 cup of boiled broccoli can meet 20% of your daily requirement of vitamin B5. The nutrients in broccoli can keep you energetic, increase your stamina, enhance immune functions, and reduce the risk of many types of cancer by 30% to 40%. They are high in antioxidants and other plant compounds that protect your body against the free radical damage and prevent developing serious diseases.

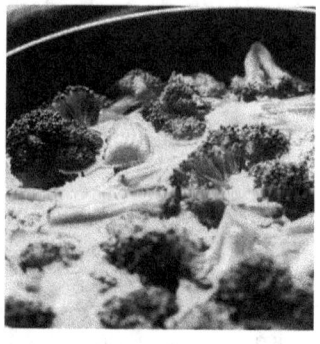

8. Chickpeas

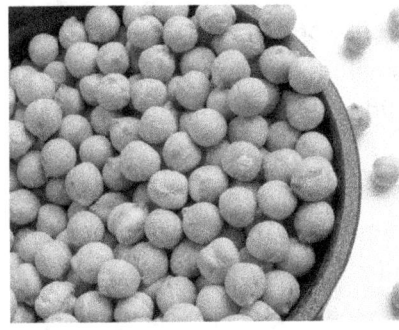

Chickpeas are another delicious way to increase your vitamin B5 consumption. 1 cup of cooked chickpeas contains 16% of the daily requirement of vitamin B5. They are a great source of fiber as they contain both soluble and insoluble fiber. Chickpeas are not only delicious but also greatly lower your bad cholesterol levels and keep your heart healthy. The fiber in chickpeas binds with cholesterol in your body and carries them out of your system. They help you feel full for a long time, reduce bad cholesterol, maintain healthy blood pressure, and prevent the onset of cardiovascular diseases.

9. Whole grains

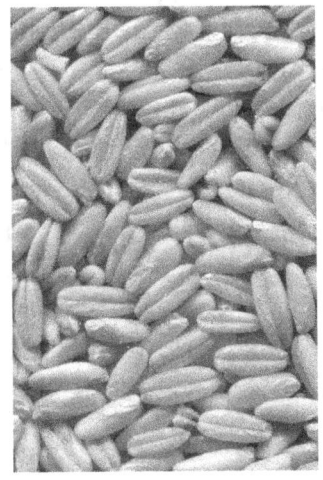

Whole grains like whole oats (oats groats), brown rice, whole wheat, and can provide you with a wealth of health benefits. The outer hard layer of the grain is the most nutrient-rich. They are hard, so they take longer to cook. During processing, this layer is removed so that the grain cooks faster, but this also reduces the nutrient density of the grain. This is why whole grains are considered healthier than refined options like white rice, refined wheat flour, and rolled oats. An easy way to use whole grains is to grind them to make flour and then use this flour in making pancakes, cakes, or chillas. 100 g of oats contain 27% daily value of vitamin B5, and 1 cup of whole wheat flour contains 12% of vitamin B5.

10. Watermelon

Watermelon keeps you cool in the summer season. It consists mainly of water; it is 90% water and is very low in calories. It is a good source of vitamins B5 and C, potassium, and magnesium. 1 cup of chopped watermelon contains 7% daily value of pantothenic acid. They are high in antioxidants like vitamin C, carotenoids, and lycopene. These antioxidants 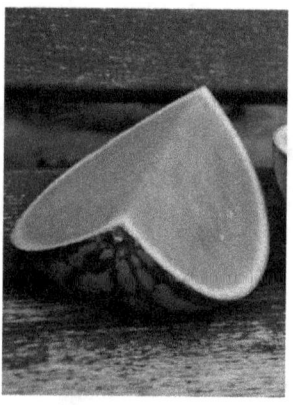 help kill free radicals in your body and prevent damage to the protein, lipids, and DNA by oxidative stress, which helps reduce your risk of chronic diseases like diabetes, neurodegenerative diseases, heart disease, and cancer.

Chapter 5
VITAMIN B6

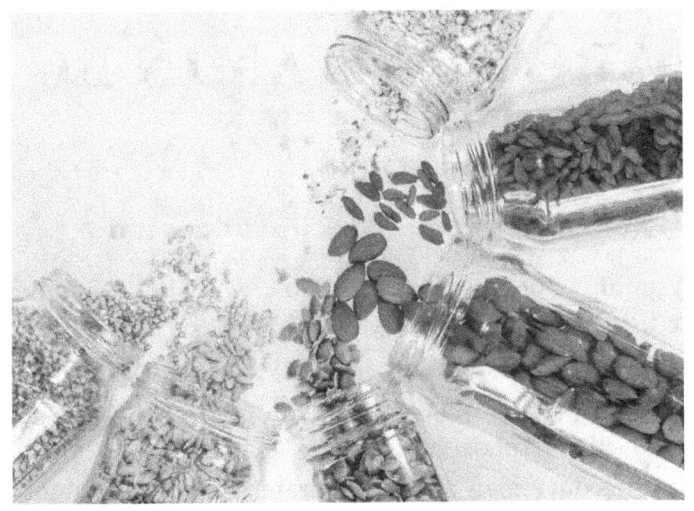

1.
EVERYTHING YOU NEED TO KNOW ABOUT VITAMIN B6

What is vitamin B6, and what does it do?

Vitamin B6 is a water-soluble essential vitamin. Vitamin B6 is the collective name for six compounds that have vitamin B6 activity: pyridoxine (PN), pyridoxal (PL), and pyridoxamine (PM) and their respective 5'-phosphate esters. Pyridoxine is essential in the conversion of carbohydrates, fats, and proteins into energy - adenosine triphosphate (ATP) - and in the production of red blood cells. It also plays an important role in maintaining cognitive health and immune function and reducing the risk of cardiovascular disease.

What are the active forms of pyridoxine?

Pyridoxal 5' phosphate (PLP) and pyridoxamine 5' phosphate (PMP) are the biologically active coenzyme forms of vitamin B6. Forms of vitamin B6 like pyridoxine, pyridoxal, and pyridoxamine and their phosphate esters are all transformed into their active forms in the body. Vitamin B6 in coenzyme forms is involved in over 100 enzyme reactions and performs various functions in your body. PLP is involved in the metabolism of carbohydrates and lipids, while both PLP and PMP are involved in protein metabolism.

How is vitamin B6 metabolized in the body?

Vitamin B6 has a high bioavailability in the body because of its good absorption from the gastrointestinal tract. Your body absorbs pyridoxine, pyridoxal, and pyridoxamine, mainly in the jejunum. The phosphorylated forms of vitamin B6 are first dephosphorylated, and then the free form of vitamin B6 is absorbed by passive diffusion. After absorption, pyridoxine is converted to its active form, coenzyme PLP (pyridoxal 5' phosphate). Dephosphorylation of PLP to PL occurs by phosphohydrolase enzymes as cell membranes are impermeable to PLP. PL is then released into the bloodstream and transported to other tissues by RBCs. Vitamin B6, or pyridoxine, is deactivated in the liver and forms inactive 4-pyridoxic acid, which is then excreted through urine. It takes 15 to 20 days for your body to eliminate vitamin B6.

Is vitamin B6 stored in the body?

Vitamin B6 is a water-soluble vitamin, it dissolves in water and is quickly excreted through urine. Your body does not store vitamin B6, so you need to get it through food every day. However, protein promotes vitamin B6 storage in the body when vitamin B6 intake is high.

When you eat high vitamin B6 food along with a high protein diet, protein favors storage of this vitamin.

Is vitamin B6 really an essential nutrient?

Yes, vitamin B6 is an essential nutrient because your body cannot make it and you must meet your body's need of vitamin B6 through food sources.

How much vitamin B6 do I need in a day?

The recommended daily intake of pyridoxine to meet the body's needs of healthy people is given below:

Age	Male	Female
Birth to 6 m	0.1 mg*	0.1 mg*
7–12 m	0.3 mg*	0.3 mg*
1–3 yrs.	0.5 mg	0.5 mg
4–8 yrs.	0.6 mg	0.6 mg
9–13 yrs.	1.0 mg	1.0 mg
14–18 yrs.	1.3 mg	1.2 mg
19–50 yrs.	1.3 mg	1.3 mg
51+ yrs.	1.7 mg	1.5 mg

*Adequate Intake (AI): Assumed level to ensure nutritional adequacy.

What factors can be responsible for pyridoxine deficiency?

Poor diet: Vitamin B6 is present in most foods in varying amounts, so vitamin B6 deficiency is unlikely in the general population due to poor diet. However, severe malnutrition can lead to vitamin B6 deficiency.

Kidney diseases: Impaired kidney function, chronic renal insufficiency, end-stage kidney diseases, and other kidney diseases can cause vitamin B6 deficiency. These diseases can reduce the absorption of vitamin B6 in the intestine.

Malabsorption: Certain disorders affect your body's ability to absorb nutrients from your food. Malabsorption can cause malnutrition even if you eat enough nutrients. Your body is unable to absorb them properly, and without proper absorption, you don't get the essential nutrients that your body uses to function properly. Diseases such as Crohn's disease, celiac disease, and ulcerative colitis reduce the absorption of vitamin B6.

Alcoholism: Alcoholics are usually at risk of nutrient deficiencies as they eat less nutrient-rich food and usually replace meals with alcohol. Also, alcohol reduces vitamin B6 absorption as well as increases its excretion, which can result in vitamin B6 deficiency.

Bariatric and metabolic surgery: Patients who undergo metabolic and bariatric surgery may suffer from vitamin B6 deficiency. Absorption of this vitamin

B6 is reduced after these surgeries which cannot be compensated by vitamin B6 supplements which can lead to deficiency in this vitamin.

Genetic disorders: Certain genetic disorders, such as homocystinuria, can cause vitamin B6 deficiency. Homocystinuria is a genetic disease that affects the metabolism of the amino acid methionine and can lead to metabolic disorders that prevent the proper absorption of vitamin B6.

Certain medications: Antiepileptic drugs can cause vitamin B6 deficiency over time. These medications increase the breakdown of vitamin B6, resulting in decreased levels of the active form of vitamin B6 in your blood.

What are the signs of vitamin B6 deficiency?

Vitamin B6 deficiency is often associated with low levels of vitamin B12 and folic acid. People who have a mild vitamin B6 deficiency usually have no symptoms or signs for months or years. Vitamin B6 deficiency can cause irritation, hearing problems, and convulsive seizures in infants. In adults, vitamin B6 deficiency is associated with the following symptoms and signs:

- Microcytic anemia (small RBCs)
- Abnormalities in your brain waves
- Confusion
- Depression
- Swollen tongue

- Cracks at the corners of the mouth or scaling on the lips
- Weakened immune system

What happens if I have a vitamin B6 deficiency?

Vitamin B6 is essential for the normal functioning of your body. Vitamin B6 deficiency causes the following ailments:

Poor cognitive health: Vitamin B6 plays a vital role in brain development and is important for keeping your nervous system healthy. It acts as a cofactor in the biosynthesis of neurotransmitters. Vitamin B6 deficiency is associated with poor cognitive function and memory.

Cardiovascular disease: Vitamin B6, along with folic acid and vitamin B12, is needed by your body to keep homocysteine levels low, which is associated with heart disease. During vitamin B6 deficiency, your body is unable to keep homocysteine levels low, increasing the risk of cardiovascular diseases.

Weak immunity: Vitamin B6 is needed for chemical reactions in the immune system. Without enough vitamin B6, your immune system cannot function efficiently, and you are at risk of infections and pathogen attacks.

Rheumatoid arthritis: Low level of vitamin B6 is associated with rheumatoid arthritis. The chronic inflammation due to rheumatoid arthritis can further reduce vitamin B6 levels and worsen the condition.

Microcytic anemia: Vitamin B6 deficiency can lead to microcytic anemia. Heme is an iron-containing molecule that combines with the globin protein to form hemoglobin. The synthesis of heme depends on the active form of vitamin B6 (PLP). Vitamin B6 deficiency reduces heme synthesis, which causes reduced hemoglobin synthesis. This leads to the production of fewer red blood cells than normal, and your organs do not get enough oxygen to function normally. This is known as microcytic anemia.

Cancer: Studies have shown that vitamin B6 helps lower the risk of certain types of cancer. Pyridoxine deficiency may increase your risk of certain types of cancer.

What if I take too much pyridoxine?

Pyridoxine is a water-soluble vitamin that is not stored in the body for long periods of time, so a high intake of vitamin B6 is not associated with any adverse effects. However, long-term (about 1 year to 3.5 years) use of high doses of about 1-6 grams of oral pyridoxine per day may cause the following adverse effects:

- Loss of control over physical movements
- Photosensitivity
- Heartburn
- Nausea
- Painful disfiguring skin lesions

These adverse effects usually disappear when the person stops taking vitamin B6 supplements.

The safe limit or upper limit for vitamin B6 below which adverse effects do not occur is 100 mg/day for adults. The upper limit for children and adolescents is lower depending on their body size. However, the upper limit may be higher for people who are advised to take vitamin B6 for their medical conditions under the supervision of a physician.

How is vitamin B6 deficiency diagnosed?

Vitamin B6 deficiency is diagnosed based on signs and symptoms, existing medical conditions that may cause the deficiency, and response to vitamin B6 supplements. The following methods are used to diagnose vitamin B6 deficiency when needed:

Direct Method

Vitamin B6 concentrations can be directly measured by assessing plasma PLP concentration or the concentration of other vitamers or total vitamin B6 in serum, plasma, or erythrocytes. The result reflects liver concentrations of vitamin B6 and is not affected by dietary fluctuations in vitamin B6 intake. The plasma PLP method is the most common measure of vitamin B6 status.

The ranges for this test are:
More than 30 nmol/l = Normal
20-30 nmol/l = Marginal deficient
Less than 20 nm/l = Deficiency

Indirect Methods

Urinary Excretion Method: This is an indirect method to measure vitamin B6 status. In this method, a 2g tryptophan load is given to the patient. After that, urinary excretion of xanthurenic acid, which is the product of tryptophan metabolism, is measured. Vitamin B6 is required for the amino acid tryptophan metabolism, and deficiency of vitamin B6 impairs tryptophan metabolism.

The ranges for urinary excretion of xanthurenic are as follows:

Less than 65 mmol/day = Normal vitamin B6 levels
More than 65 mmol/day = Abnormal tryptophan metabolism due to vitamin B6 insufficiency.

To indicate adequate short-term vitamin B6 status, urinary excretion of 4-pyridoxic acid is measured which is reported as urinary pyridoxic acid.

More than 3.0 mmol/day urinary excretion of 4-pyridoxic acid indicates adequate levels of vitamin B6 in the body

Erythrocyte Transaminase Activity: Vitamin B6 levels can also be measured indirectly by assessing erythrocyte aminotransferase saturation by PLP. It is a functional test of vitamin B6 levels which is more accurate reflection of vitamin B6 levels in critically ill patients

2. IMPORTANCE OF VITAMIN B6

The biologically active form of vitamin B6, pyridoxal phosphate (PLP), is an important coenzyme. It is needed by more than a hundred enzymes that catalyze chemical reactions vital to your body's normal function. Some of the most important enzymatically catalyzed chemical reactions that depend on PLP as a coenzyme are described below.

FUNCTIONS OF PYRIDOXINE IN THE BODY

Energy Production

Like other B vitamins, vitamin B6 is required for energy production from dietary proteins, carbohydrates, and fats. The active forms of vitamin B6 participate mainly in protein metabolism. The vitamin B6 derivatives pyridoxal phosphate (PLP) and pyridoxamine phosphate (PMP) are involved in amino acid metabolism, while pyridoxal phosphate also participates in carbohydrate and fat metabolism.

Formation of Vitamin B3 in the Body

Niacin or vitamin B3 can be formed from the breakdown of an essential amino acid tryptophan. Adequate levels of PLP help maintain the formation of vitamin B3 from tryptophan in the body. Without enough vitamin B6, your body cannot convert tryptophan into NAD, the active form of vitamin B3. Tryptophan metabolism through the kynurenine pathway produces several biologically active intermediate metabolites. One branch of the kynurenine pathway leads to the synthesis of NAD- nicotinamide adenine dinucleotide, the active form of vitamin B3. The synthesis of niacin from tryptophan requires PLP-dependent enzymes that catalyze this reaction. PLP acts as a cofactor for the enzyme that facilitates the formation of niacin. A deficiency in vitamin B6 affects the metabolism of tryptophan to niacin.

Maintain Normal Homocysteine Levels

Even a moderate increase in homocysteine levels in your blood is dangerous to your health. High homocysteine levels in your blood are associated with increased risks of myocardial infarction, heart attack, and stroke. Methionine, an essential amino released during protein metabolism, is required for methylation reactions such as methylation of proteins, DNA, and RNA. The metabolism of methionine forms an intermediate called homocysteine, which, if not broken down, can increase the risk of cardiovascular diseases and stroke.

Homocysteine levels can be reduced in two ways: either it is remethylated to methionine, which requires vitamin B9 and vitamin B12, or it can be broken down into another essential amino acid, cysteine, which your body uses to make proteins and antioxidants like glutathione. Converting homocysteine to cysteine requires two enzymes that need the active metabolite of vitamin B6 (PLP) to function. Without enough vitamin B6 in your body, homocysteine cannot be broken down, and its blood levels increase, significantly increasing your risk of cardiovascular and cerebrovascular diseases.

Formation of Hemoglobin

Hemoglobin is the primary part of your red blood cells that enables them to carry oxygen. The quality of hemoglobin affects the formation of red blood cells. Vitamin B6 is important in the formation of hemoglobin and is required for the production of normal red blood cells. Pyridoxine is involved in the conversion of iron into hemoglobin. The biologically active form of pyridoxine, pyridoxal 5'-phosphate (PLP), is involved in the first enzymatic step in heme synthesis. PLP acts as a cofactor for the 5'-aminolevulinic acid synthase (ALA-S), the first enzyme in heme synthesis. Both pyridoxal and the active metabolite PLP can bind to hemoglobin and affect its ability to pick up oxygen and release it to tissues in your body.

Immune Function

Low levels of pyridoxine are associated with poor immune response. Vitamin B6 is important for immune function. The metabolites of vitamin B6 are needed in chemical reactions in the immune system. It aids in the production of antibodies that help fight bacteria, viruses, infections, toxins, and other diseases. Vitamin B6 promotes the production of lymphocytes and interleukin-2. Lymphocytes are a type of white blood cell found in your immune system. Antibodies are produced by B cells, which are a type of lymphocyte. Interleukin-2 enhances the function of T-cells, natural killer cells (NK cells), and B-cells.

Essential for Glucose Homeostasis

Your body maintains normal blood sugar levels in response to internal and external conditions changes. This process is called glucose homeostasis. There are two processes through which glucose levels in the body are regulated:

Gluconeogenesis: When your diet is lacking in carbohydrates and your body does not get carbohydrates as its main source of energy, it makes glucose from other non-carbohydrate compounds such as amino acids, lactic acid, and glycerol. These reactions take place in your liver and kidneys and are called gluconeogenesis.

Glycogenolysis: When you eat a high-carbohydrate meal, your body breaks it down into glucose and converts it into energy to meet its needs. Your body stores any excess carbohydrates that are not needed at that moment as glycogen in your liver. In the case of fasting, when blood sugar levels drop and the immediate source of energy, carbohydrates, is not available, your body breaks down glycogen into glucose to provide immediate energy. This process is called glycogenolysis.

Vitamin B6, in its active form, is involved in both glycogenolysis and gluconeogenesis processes and helps maintain stable blood sugar levels.

Production of Neurotransmitters

Vitamin B6 is critical for your brain health and may protect you from cognitive decline, memory loss, and dementia. It plays an important role in the synthesis of neurotransmitters in your brain, which are important chemical substances that enable nerve cells to communicate with each other. Since vitamin B6 is involved in energy production, it increases the supply of energy to the brain, which keeps it functional and healthy. Enzymes involved in synthesizing two major neurotransmitters in the brain, dopamine from L-dopa and serotonin from the amino acid tryptophan, require PLP to perform their functions. PLP also facilitates the conversion of the neurotransmitter glutamate, which is responsible for causing excitement, into GABA neurotransmitter, an inhibitory neurotransmitter that causes a calming effect.

Anti-Inflammatory and Antioxidant Properties

Inflammation and oxidation are two processes that, when beyond normal limits, are the major cause of many chronic diseases and affect lifestyle. Both processes are important for the normal functioning of your body. They help fight pathogens and reduce the risk of infections. However, uncontrolled inflammation starts attacking your body cells and causes rheumatoid arthritis, inflammatory bowel disease, and heart disease. Oxidative stress occurs when free radicals exceed the antioxidants in the body, bind with cells in the DNA and proteins, and damage them.

Vitamin B6 has both anti-inflammatory and antioxidant properties. It prevents inflammation and kills free radicals before they can damage the body. Vitamin B6 in the PLP form helps reduce inflammatory cytokine levels by affecting the kynurenine pathway. PLP acts as a co-factor and is essential in the amino acid tryptophan metabolism. L-kynurenine hydrolase (KYNU) is a PLP-dependent enzyme; it requires PLP to function. PLP increases KYNU, which reduces inflammatory cytokine levels and thus reduces inflammation.

Vitamin B6 contributes to your body's antioxidant defense through direct and indirect pathways. Vitamin B6 can neutralize free radicals by directly reacting with peroxy radicals and preventing the oxidation of lipids. Vitamin B6 as PLP participates in the glutathione antioxidant defense system. PLP is needed as a coenzyme in the breakdown of homocysteine to cysteine. The essential amino acid cysteine is required to synthesize reduced glutathione (GSH), which is fundamental to your body's defense system. It is a natural antioxidant that prevents oxidative damage by killing free radicals and helps maintain your internal integrity.

TOP HEALTH BENEFITS OF VITAMIN B6

1. Prevent Anemia: The formation of normal, healthy, and adequate red blood cells in your body ensures the functionality of your organs. RBCs are responsible for delivering nutrients and oxygen to all your tissues and organs. Hemoglobin is an important component of RBCs; any abnormality in hemoglobin affects RBC formation. Vitamin B6 increases the production of hemoglobin, as this vitamin is crucially involved in the heme formation of hemoglobin. Eating enough vitamin B6 through diet helps prevent a type of anemia called microcytic anemia, which is primarily caused by vitamin B6 deficiency and is characterized by smaller-than-normal red blood cells because they do not contain enough hemoglobin.

2. Prevent Cardiovascular Diseases: Keeping homocysteine levels low is the key to a healthy heart. High levels of homocysteine promote atherosclerosis. Homocysteine can damage your blood vessels and increase your risk of clot formation inside your arteries, which is called a thrombus. It also increases oxidative stress, which further increases your risk of blood vessel blockage. Consuming enough vitamin B6 through dietary sources helps prevent cardiovascular diseases. Consuming enough vitamin B6 ensures that homocysteine levels remain low as it breaks homocysteine into other essential amino acids that boost your health.

3. Prevent Cancer: Vitamin B6 in the diet is associated with a reduced risk of breast, stomach, esophageal and colorectal cancer. Vitamin B6 is involved in various chemical reactions in the body and supports a wide range of cellular functions; therefore, it prevents cancer in many ways. Vitamin B6 helps prevent oxidative damage to DNA by acting as an antioxidant agent and promoting the synthesis of other antioxidants in your body. Vitamin B6, along with folate and B12, is involved in one-carbon metabolism, which is an important pathway for the synthesis of DNA and is essential for DNA repair and cell proliferation. Vitamin B6 also prevents the formation of DNA damaging advanced glycation end products (AGEs).

4. Prevent Neurodegenerative Diseases: Vitamin B6 can boost your cognitive health and reduce your risk of neurodegenerative diseases like Alzheimer's disease, Parkinson's disease, and dementia. High levels of homocysteine in the body are linked to stroke as it damages blood vessels and blocks the normal flow of blood to the brain. Pyridoxine helps maintain normal levels of homocysteine. It also plays a critical role in the biosynthesis of neurotransmitters like dopamine, melatonin, serotonin, etc., which help your brain function at its best. Getting enough dopamine can help prevent Parkinson's disease.

5. Manage Premenstrual Syndrome: Vitamin B6 is great for menstruating women. Vitamin B6 can make your premenstrual days easier. Consuming adequate amounts of vitamin B6 through diet helps reduce premenstrual symptoms as well as prevent mood fluctuations associated with periods. It has anti-inflammatory properties that help reduce pain and swelling. Also, it increases several mood-enhancing neurotransmitters in your brain and helps calm you down. It may not be effective in relieving cramps, but it can definitely improve your mood, reduce irritability, relieve fatigue, and prevent depressive feelings.

6. Boost Immunity: Vitamin B6 helps boost your immunity. High vitamin B6 intake through dietary sources is associated with better immune function as it is involved in various chemical reactions of the immune system. With vitamin B6, you can fight infections better. Vitamin B6 helps produce antibodies that protect you from bacterial and viral infections. When unwanted substances enter your body, these antibodies bind to the foreign bodies and flush them out of your system.

7. Prevent Eye Diseases: Age-related macular degeneration (AMD) is a common reason for vision loss in old age. High levels of homocysteine and free radicals are directly associated with an increased risk of AMD. Vitamin B6 significantly reduces circulating levels of homocysteine, which helps reduce the risk of this disease. In addition, vitamin B6 supports your body's antioxidant defense system and the biosynthesis of essential antioxidants that help deactivate free radicals, prevent oxidative damage to your eyes, and promote eye health.

8. Prevent Nausea in Pregnancy: Pyridoxine has many roles in ensuring a healthy pregnancy. A vitamin B6-rich diet can prevent nausea and severe morning sickness during pregnancy. It is used medically to treat nausea and vomiting in pregnancy. A high vitamin B6 diet also increases the immune tolerance of the baby. However, it's crucial to consult your physician before taking vitamin B6 supplements.

3.
10 RICHEST VEGETARIAN SOURCES OF VITAMIN B6

Below are top 10 vegetarian sources of Vitamin B6 (Pyridoxine):

1. Chickpeas

Chickpeas are one of the best sources of vitamin B6 or

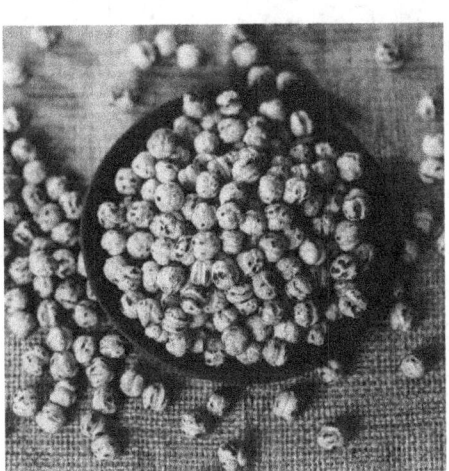

pyridoxine. One cup of cooked chickpeas fulfills 65% of your daily requirement of vitamin B6. They are a great source of protein, fiber, potassium and magnesium.

Chickpeas control your blood pressure greatly due to

their high potassium and magnesium content. Also, the high fiber in chickpeas removes cholesterol from your body. Low blood pressure and low cholesterol levels in your body help keep your heart healthy and prevent heart attacks.

2. Sweet Potato

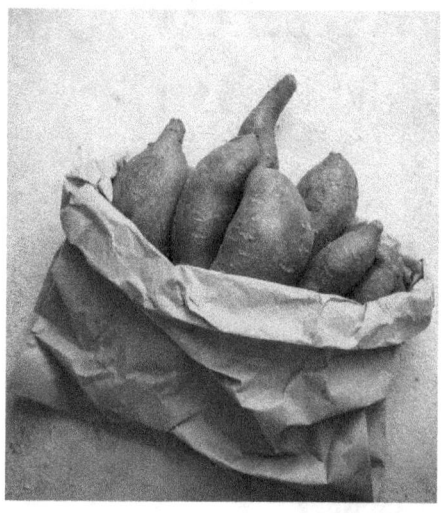

Sweet potato is considered a superfood due to its dense nutrient content. It is loaded with a variety of vitamins and minerals. It is a good source of vitamin B6. 1 cup of boiled sweet potato contains 32% of the daily value of vitamin B6. It is also a great source of vitamin A and dietary fiber. It is lower in glycemic index than white potatoes and releases sugar slowly into the blood which helps in diabetes management. Vitamin A in sweet potato acts as an antioxidant and protects you from eye disorders by minimizing oxidative stress in your body.

3. Banana

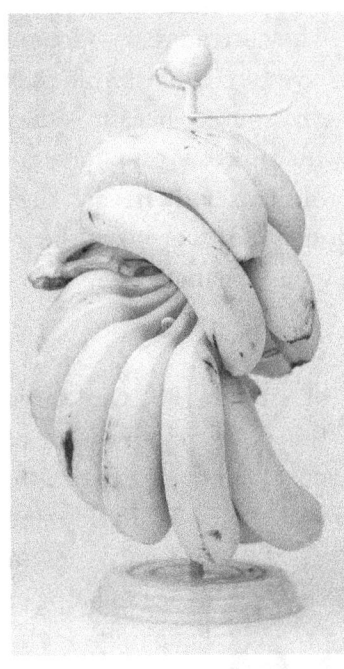

Both ripe and green bananas are good sources of vitamin B6. Eat a banana before leaving home, it will keep you energetic and suppress your unnecessary sudden hunger. It is good for sports people to provide instant energy. It helps in controlling blood pressure as it contains a good amount of potassium which helps in balancing sodium in your body and keeps your heart healthy. Bananas also help in improving mood. Eating banana as a snack can instantly improve your mood and make you feel full of energy. A medium-sized banana can provide you 25% of daily value of vitamin B6.

4. Soybean

Soybeans are an excellent source of pyridoxine as well as other B vitamins and fat-soluble vitamins. 1 cup of cooked soybeans can meet 24% of your daily requirement of vitamin B6. They are a great source of protein and potassium and have zero cholesterol. They are the high-quality protein source because they contain complete protein which means they have all the nine amino acids that a human body needs. They help prevent the development of coronary heart disease, stroke, and certain types of cancer.

5. Avocado

Avocado is a good source of vitamin B6. One large avocado contains 30% of the daily requirement of vitamin B6. Avocado helps boost your cognitive health.

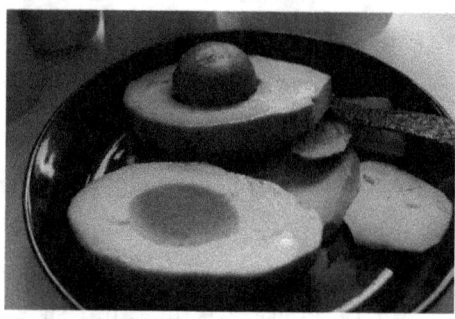

Pyridoxine present in avocado helps in keeping the homocysteine levels in the body normal and thus prevents the development of cardiovascular diseases. It increases the hemoglobin levels in your body which ensures that nutrient-rich and oxygen-filled blood reaches every tissue and organ of the body and thus protects the functioning of your organs.

6. Nuts

Nuts are a good source of vitamin B6, especially pistachios and sunflower seeds. A handful (about 28 grams) of pistachios can provide you with 28% of the daily value of vitamin B6, and a handful of sunflower seeds meet 22% of your daily requirement of vitamin B6. In addition, they are a good source of other B vitamins and healthy fats that help keep

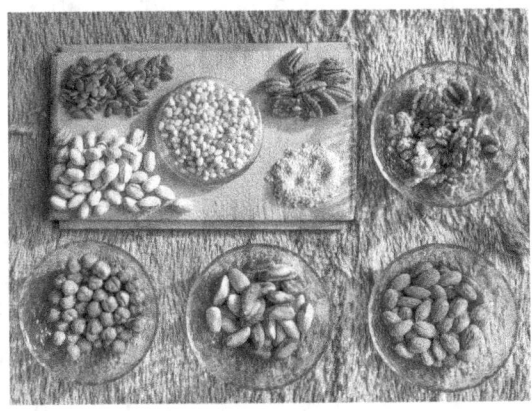

your body's cellular function normal. They boost your immune health, keep your nerves healthy, and ultimately enhance your brain health.

7. Bulgur/Dalia

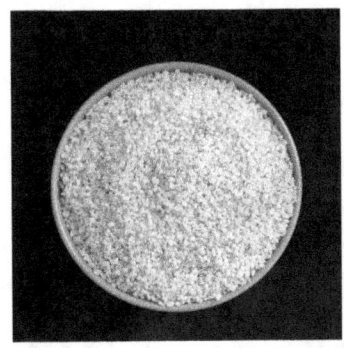

Bulgur or Daliya is the cracked whole wheat. It is easy to cook and digest. Since the germ and bran layers are not removed from bulgur, it retains most of the vitamins and minerals that are not present in refined wheat. The high fiber content of bulgur aids digestion and promotes weight loss. It helps control diabetes and prevent cardiovascular disorders. They are packed with important vitamins and minerals. 1 cup of bulgur contains 28% of the daily value of vitamin B6. It has high magnesium and iron content that promotes your brain health and enhances your cognitive power.

8. Mango

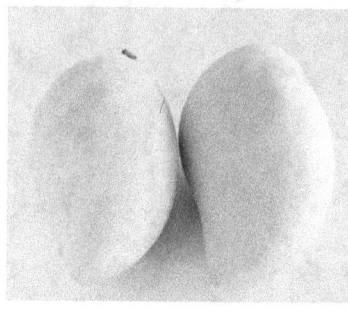

Mangoes are an excellent source of vitamin B6. One large mango (about 335 grams) contains 39% of your daily recommended intake of pyridoxine. Mangoes are rich in antioxidants, and plant compounds called polyphenols. These polyphenols are protectors in plants that protect plants from the invasion of pathogens. Similarly, when these polyphenols are consumed by humans, they produce similar effects. They protect against pathogens and prevent the onset of various diseases. They are good for digestion and reduce constipation. They promote brain health by keeping your nerve cells healthy.

9. Rice

Rice is a good source of pyridoxine. Both brown rice and white rice provide adequate amounts of vitamin B6. Many nutrients are removed while polishing white rice; however,

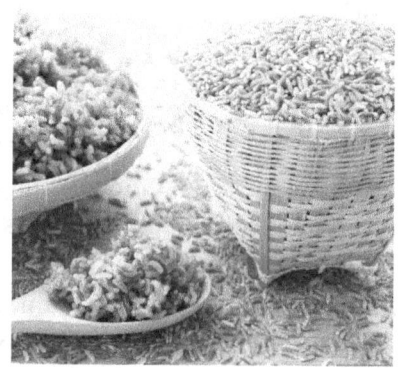

manufacturers usually add the lost nutrients back into the rice. Choose brown rice over white rice for maximum health benefits. Brown rice contains many naturally occurring vitamins and minerals that are not found in fortified white rice. They help reduce your risk of diabetes and cancer and promote heart health. They keep the digestive system healthy. The high B vitamins in rice provide you with consistent energy and keep your organs working efficiently. 1 cup of cooked brown rice has a 15% daily value of vitamin B6.

10. Carrots

Carrots are a fair source of vitamin B6. 1 cup of chopped carrots can meet 10% of your daily vitamin B6 requirement. Vitamin B6 is not heat sensitive, so cooking or baking carrots does not affect their vitamin B6

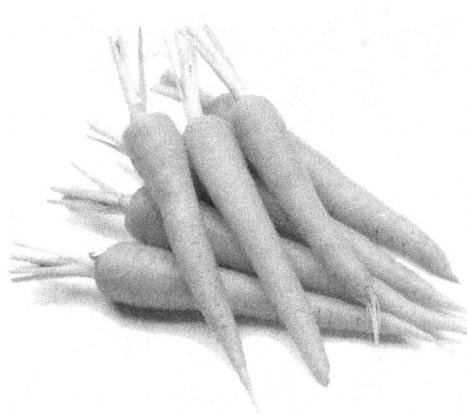

content. You can eat them raw, make a puree or soup, or add them to your noodles. Carrots have a high-water content, which makes them good for weight management. They promote your eye health, reduce your risk of cancer, lower blood pressure and blood sugar, and keep your heart healthy.

Chapter 6
VITAMIN B7

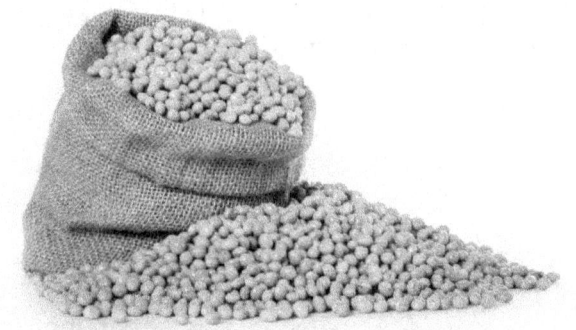

1.
EVERYTHING YOU NEED TO KNOW ABOUT VITAMIN B7

What is vitamin B7 and what does it do?

Vitamin B7 is also known as biotin, which is an essential water-soluble nutrient that you need to obtain from food. Biotin acts as a cofactor for five carboxylase enzymes in your body that participate in various steps in the metabolism of fats, glucose, and amino acids. Your body also needs biotin for gene regulation and cell signaling. Other names for vitamin B7 are vitamin H and coenzyme R.

What are the five carboxylases that need biotin as a cofactor?

What are the five carboxylases that require biotin as a cofactor? The five carboxylase enzymes for which biotin acts as a cofactor are acetyl-CoA carboxylase 1, acetyl-CoA carboxylase 2, propionyl-CoA carboxylase, methylcrotonyl-CoA carboxylase (MCC), and pyruvate carboxylase.

How is vitamin B7 metabolized in the body?

Biotin in food is mostly bound to proteins, but some foods contain free biotin. When you consume a biotin-rich food, your gastric enzymes, such as protease and peptidase, break down biotin-protein-bound into biocytin and biotin-oligopeptides. An enzyme called biotinidase breaks down biocytin and biotin-oligopeptides, releasing free biotin into the intestinal lumen. The free biotin is then absorbed in your small intestine.

Is vitamin B7 stored in my body?

Biotin is a water-soluble vitamin, so it dissolves in water and is readily excreted through urine, and does not stay in your system for long. This means that, unlike fat-soluble vitamins, biotin is not stored well in your body. The biotin you consume is excreted from your system within 72 hours, and most of the biotin is stored in your liver.

Is vitamin B7 really an essential nutrient?

Your gut bacteria can make some biotin, however, this amount is not enough to meet your body's needs, which is why biotin is considered an essential vitamin that you must obtain from food sources to meet your body's biotin needs.

How much vitamin B7 do I need a day?

There is not enough data available to establish the RDA, i.e., Recommended Dietary Allowances, so the AI is established. The adequate intake or AI is established when data is insufficient to establish an RDA that represents sufficient intake levels to ensure nutritional adequacy and prevent nutrient deficiencies. The adequate intake of biotin for most healthy people is given below:

Age	Male	Female
Birth to 6 m	5 mcg	5 mcg
7–12 m	6 mcg	6 mcg
1–3 yrs.	8 mcg	8 mcg
4–8 yrs.	12 mcg	12 mcg
9–13 yrs.	20 mcg	20 mcg
14–18 yrs.	25 mcg	25 mcg
19+ yrs.	30 mcg	30 mcg

What factors can be responsible for biotin deficiency?

Biotin deficiency is very rare. However, the following conditions can cause insufficient levels of biotin in your body:

Consuming raw eggs: Consuming raw eggs in mayonnaise, eggnog, Caesar dressing, etc., can lead to biotin deficiency. Raw eggs contain avidin, a protein that prevents the absorption of biotin in your body by forming a complex with biotin. Since your body cannot break down avidin, the biotin bound to avidin passes out of your body without being absorbed, and you do not get the benefits of biotin, leading to its deficiency. When you cook eggs, the avidin protein is broken down due to the heat, making it easier to digest and allowing your body to absorb the biotin easily.

Ketogenic diet: The keto diet is high in fat and low in carbohydrates. This causes your body to break down fat into ketones, which are used as energy. The keto diet is often linked to biotin deficiency. Biotin is involved in fatty acid metabolism; the ketogenic diet increases biotin consumption for energy production which leads to biotin deficiency in your body.

Biotinidase deficiency: Biotinidase deficiency is a rare genetic condition in which the body is unable to release free biotin, leading to biotin deficiency even if the person has a normal intake of biotin.

Smoking: Smoking increases the breakdown of biotin, which leads to reduced biotin content in the body.

Alcohol addiction: Alcohol inhibits the absorption of biotin as well as interferes with its metabolism, resulting in biotin deficiency. Alcoholics generally have a poor diet and replace meals with alcohol, which further increases the risk of biotin deficiency.

Certain diseases: Certain conditions, such as Crohn's disease and celiac disease, prevent the normal absorption of vitamin B7 in your body, which can lead to biotin deficiency.

Certain medicines: Long-term use of certain medications, such as antiseizure medications and antibiotics, affects your body's absorption of biotin, which can lead to biotin deficiency. Long-term use of antibiotics causes changes in the gut flora, which negatively affects the production of biotin by the gut flora, which contributes to inadequate levels of biotin in your body.

Pregnancy and nursing: Pregnant women often suffer from biotin deficiency, similarly biotin deficiency is also found in nursing mothers. The exact reason behind this is not yet known. If a pregnant woman or nursing mother is deficient in biotin, it can cause vitamin B7 deficiency in the baby. Therefore, talk to your doctor for any necessary biotin supplements, do not take them yourself, consult a healthcare provider to adjust the dosage.

What are the signs and symptoms of Vitamin B7 deficiency?

The signs and symptoms of biotin deficiency are as follows:

- Thinning hair which can lead to loss (alopecia)
- Scaly dry skin
- Red rashes around eyes, mouth, and nose
- Brittle nails
- Conjunctivitis
- Depression
- Hallucinations

- Fatigue
- Insomnia

What happens if I am deficient in biotin?

Vitamin B7 deficiency can lead to the following conditions:

Biotin deficient facies: Biotin deficiency leads to impaired fatty acid metabolism, which can cause skin abnormalities like facial rashes with abnormal fat distribution on the face, which is termed as biotin deficient facies.

Hair loss (alopecia): Vitamin B7 is essential for the health of your hair. Biotin helps prevent hair thinning and split ends. This is why it is used along with zinc in the treatment of alopecia. Biotin deficiency can lead to hair loss.

Improper development of the baby: Biotin deficiency during pregnancy can cause growth retardation, developmental delay and congenital malformation in babies.

Cradle cap: Babies who don't have enough biotin may develop thick, yellow, scaly patches on their scalp.

Seborrheic dermatitis: Biotin deficiency can lead to seborrheic dermatitis, which is characterized by greasy scales and red itchy patches on your skin.

Conjunctivitis: Biotin is involved in enzymatic reactions that are important for maintaining the health of your eyes. Biotin deficiency can cause eye problems such as conjunctivitis.

Skin Infections: Biotin is essential for good skin. Biotin is involved in fatty acid metabolism. Biotin deficiency adversely affects the immune system and fat metabolism, putting you at increased risk of skin infections.

Lactic Acidosis: Lactic acidosis is characterized by the build-up of lactic acid in the bloodstream. It occurs when the rate of lactate production exceeds the rate of lactate clearance from your body. Biotin deficiency causes decreased activity of biotin-dependent carboxylase enzymes. Decreased activity of the pyruvate carboxylase enzyme leads to lactic acidosis.

Ketoacidosis and organic aciduria: Biotin deficiency reduces the activity of biotin-dependent carboxylase enzymes, which affects the levels of various intermediate metabolites, leading to metabolic errors such as organic aciduria and ketoacidosis. Organic aciduria is characterized by the accumulation of toxic abnormal organic acid metabolites in the blood and increased excretion of these in the urine. Ketoacidosis is characterized by the accumulation of ketone bodies in the blood and increased excretion of these in the urine.

What happens if I take too much biotin?

Biotin does not cause any toxicity in your body. It is a water-soluble vitamin, so any excess biotin is excreted in the urine. Excess biotin from natural sources is safe; however, excess biotin through dietary supplements can cause some side effects, including excessive thirst, urination, and insomnia. Biotin is involved in glucose control, so excess biotin causes symptoms of hyperglycemia. Therefore, people with diabetes should consult their doctor before taking biotin supplements.

How is vitamin B7 deficiency diagnosed?

Biotin deficiency is rare. Therefore, very limited sensitive indicators of biotin status are available.

Blood Test: Serum concentration of 133-329 pmol/L indicates normal biotin levels in your body.

Urine Test: Urine excretion of 18-127 nmol/24 hours indicates healthy biotin levels.

Less than 18 nmol in 24 hours indicates low levels of biotin.

Excretion of biotin metabolites, 3-hydroxyisovaleric acid of more than 3.3 mmol/mol creatinine, or excretion of 3-hydroxyisovalerylcarnitine more than 0.06 mmol/mol creatinine indicates low activity of the biotin-dependent enzyme methylcrotonyl-CoA carboxylase (MCC).

2.
IMPORTANCE OF VITAMIN B7

FUNCTIONS OF BIOTIN IN THE BODY

Gluconeogenesis

Gluconeogenesis is the process through which your body makes glucose from non-carbohydrate substrates such as lactate, glycerol pyruvate, and propionate. When you fast or you do not consume enough carbohydrates to convert into energy, your body breaks down other non-carbohydrate substrates into glucose so that your body can generate enough energy to function properly. Biotin has an important role in gluconeogenesis and helps maintain normal glucose levels in your body. Biotin plays the role of a cofactor for the enzyme pyruvate carboxylase. Biotin-dependent pyruvate carboxylase converts pyruvate into oxaloacetate, which is necessary for the initial step in gluconeogenesis.

Fatty Acid Synthesis

Biotin acts as a cofactor for carboxylase enzymes. They are called carboxylase enzymes because they add a carboxylic acid group to the compound they work on. Your body makes fatty acids such as saturated fatty acids, unsaturated fatty acids, and triglycerides to be used for signaling functions and as energy sources in case glucose is unavailable. When you have excess carbohydrates in your body, even after meeting your body's energy requirements, the excess glucose is converted into pyruvate through glycolysis. Pyruvate is converted into acetyl-CoA. Acetyl-CoA is then converted to malonyl CoA, and the enzyme that catalyzes this conversion requires biotin to perform its function. After a few more steps, saturated fatty acid molecules are produced, which can be desaturated to form unsaturated fatty acids. Without enough biotin, these reactions cannot continue, which disrupts your body's internal integrity.

Branch-Chain Amino Acids (BCAA) Catabolism

Branch-chain amino acid catabolism plays an essential role in regulating glucose metabolism. Biotin is important as a cofactor of carboxylase enzymes such as propionyl-CoA carboxylase, which is involved in the catabolism of many branch-chain amino acids and β-methylcrotonyl-CoA carboxylase, which is required for the catabolism of leucine. The catabolism of branch-chain amino acids yields chemicals that further participate in other reactions and are important for ensuring the normal functioning of your body.

Histone Modification

Histones are proteins that provide structural support for the chromosome. They mediate the folding of DNA into chromatin. Biotin is involved in histone modification. The enzyme biotinidase mediates biotin binding to histones, which is called biotinylation. Histone modifications are associated with increased DNA transcription, replication, and repair mechanisms that influence the effects of acetylation, ADP-ribosylation, and phosphorylation of histones. These are essential for maintaining the integrity of DNA, protecting DNA from damage, and influencing immune responses.

Keratin Formation

Keratin is a fibrous protein that is a major structural protein in hair and nails and forms the outermost skin barrier. Biotin plays a vital role in the formation of keratin and the structuring and improvement of the health of skin, hair, and nails. Keratin proteins are the protective matrix of the skin, hair, and nails. The formation of keratin proteins involves the transformation of living, highly functional skin cells into dead but structurally stable cells with no biological activity. Adequate availability of biotin, along with other nutrients, determines the quality and integrity of keratin formation. Eating enough biotin-rich foods produces healthy and strong hair, nails, and skin.

TOP HEALTH BENEFITS OF VITAMIN B7

1. Prevent and Reverse Hair Loss: Biotin deficiency causes hair loss. It promotes keratin production in your body, and your hair is primarily made of keratin. Biotin is used in various hair products; however, research studies on biotin preventing hair loss have shown mixed results. Biotin intake can prevent and reverse hair loss if the cause of hair loss is insufficient biotin levels. Consuming enough biotin can nourish your hair follicles, reducing hair loss, preventing split ends, and promoting smooth, shiny, and healthy hair.

2. Promote Healthy Pregnancy: Biotin is an important vitamin during pregnancy. Vitamin B7 is involved in histone modification and plays various important biological roles in a healthy pregnancy, such as immune function and fetal development. Biotin is essential for the normal growth and development of the baby. It enhances cognitive health and immune functions and prevents cradle cap, a type of scalp condition characterized by thick and scaly patches on the baby's scalp.

3. Treat Ageusia (Loss of Taste): Ageusia is a rare condition in which a person completely loses the taste function of the tongue. Loss of taste is distressing and negatively affects the quality of life. Research has proven that biotin has a positive relationship with taste. Vitamin B7 successfully helps restore taste in people who have lost the sense of taste for no apparent reason.

4. Seborrheic Dermatitis: Biotin deficiency can cause seborrheic dermatitis in infants as well as adults. Seborrheic dermatitis is characterized by red, greasy scaly patches that occur on the area where there are a lot of sebum-producing sebaceous glands, such as the scalp, around the nose, outer ears, and between the nose and upper lips. Consuming a diet rich in biotin is quite effective in treating seborrheic dermatitis, as biotin blocks the main metabolic pathways that lead to the development of seborrheic dermatitis.

5. Peripheral Neuropathy: Biotin is beneficial in improving peripheral neuropathy, a nerve disease in which the nerve cells outside the brain and spinal cord are damaged. Long-term treatment with vitamin B7 improves symptoms of peripheral neuropathy such as speech disorders, disorientation, memory loss, restless legs, and difficulty in walking.

6. Manage Diabetes: Biotin may help control blood sugar levels, especially in people with diabetes. Biotin corrects glucose metabolism in diabetes. It increases the activity of the biotin-dependent carboxylase enzyme, pyruvate, and promotes the use of glucose for energy production. It also regulates insulin-releasing beta-cell function in the pancreas and increases the potency of insulin action, which helps keep blood sugar low.

7. Cognitive Health: Vitamin B7 is a neuroprotective agent. It protects the health of nerve cells. It regulates cell signals and promotes fast and efficient communication throughout your body. Biotin plays an essential role in the metabolism of glucose in your brain. It regulates the absorption of glucose in the liver and maintains glucose hemostasis. Your brain is essentially sensitive to the delivery and metabolism of glucose. Biotin maintains a constant energy supply to the brain and keeps its nerve cells healthy. Additionally, biotin has antioxidant activity and helps reduce oxidative stress biomarkers in your brain, which protects the integrity of your nerve cells and prevents memory loss, dementia, and Alzheimer's disease.

8. Healthy Skin and Nails: Biotin is a vital nutrient for maintaining skin health. It supports the synthesis of fatty acids, which are essential for maintaining skin integrity. It also helps maintain the function of oil glands, which nourish the skin, form a protective layer, and prevent skin damage.

Vitamin B7-rich foods help treat brittle nails. It increases the formation of a protein called keratin. Your nails are made up of keratin protein. Biotin strengthens your nails and increases their hardness, thickness, and firmness.

3.
10 RICHEST VEGETARIAN SOURCES OF VITAMIN B7

Below are the 10 richest vegetarian sources of Vitamin B7 (Biotin):

1. Walnut

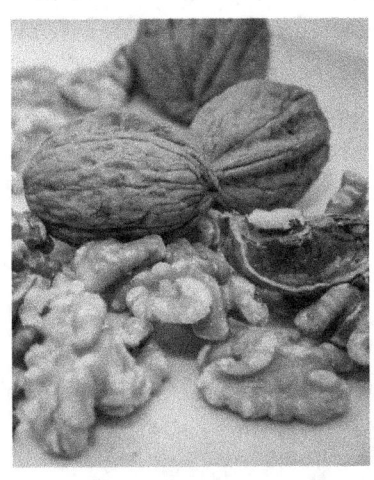

Walnuts are the best source of biotin. A handful of walnuts (30 grams) contains 37% of the daily requirement of biotin. They are also a great source of alpha-linolenic acid, vitamin E, monounsaturated fats, copper, and manganese. Walnuts are great for your hair and heart health. Inflammation is the major cause of many chronic diseases, including but not limited to rheumatoid arthritis, diabetes, cancer, and heart disease. Walnuts help reduce inflammation in your body and prevent cholesterol build-up, which causes heart diseases.

2. Soybeans

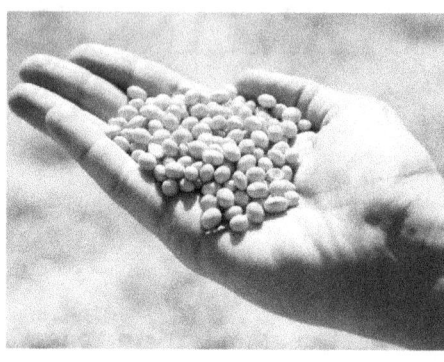

Soybeans are an excellent source of biotin. ¾ cup of cooked soybeans can meet 64% of your daily biotin requirement. The high biotin in soybeans promotes liver health and hair growth and boosts your memory. Soybeans are also an excellent source of other essential nutrients such as thiamine, folate, vitamin K1, copper, phosphorus, and manganese. The high protein in soybeans keeps you full for a long time and prevents unnecessary cravings which helps in weight management.

3. Amaranth

Amaranth plants are classified as pseudo-cereals. This is because they fall under the category of cereals but they are not true grains like wheat and rice, they are actually seeds

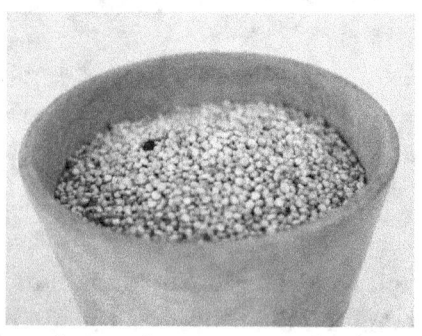

not grains. Since they provide the same nutrients as whole grains they are considered grains. Also, they are gluten free unlike most grains. Amaranth seeds contain a good amount of biotin. 100 grams of amaranth seeds contain 54% of your daily requirement of vitamin B7. You can easily make amaranth flour from amaranth at home and mix it with your chapati dough and tortilla four.

4. Mushrooms

Several varieties of mushrooms, like button mushrooms, portabella, and cremini mushrooms, are

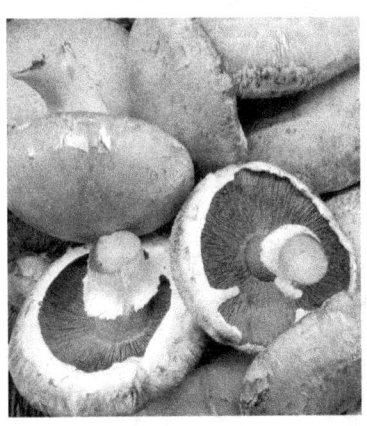

rich sources of vitamin B7. They contain important nutrients for healthy hair. The selenium present in mushrooms supports healthy hair follicles, promotes thicker and stronger hair, and prevents hair loss. Selenium, along with biotin, works wonders for your hair and prevents split ends and dry and brittle hair. Mushrooms are low in calories and can be a good source of vitamin D, which is usually not present in a vegetarian diet. 100 g of cooked button mushrooms fulfill 27% of your body's daily requirement of biotin. Similarly, 100 grams of portabella mushrooms fulfill 37% of the daily requirement of biotin.

5. Peanuts

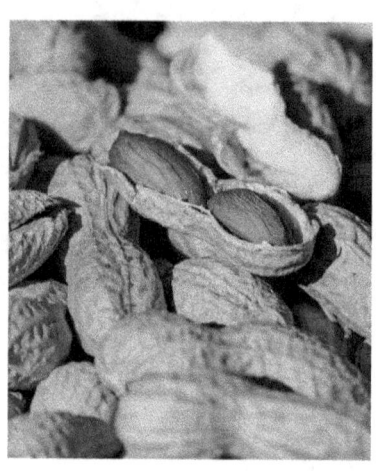

Peanuts are one of the best sources of biotin. A handful of roasted peanuts (about 28 grams) can meet 17% of daily value of biotin and keep your skin, hair, nails, and brain healthy. Peanuts are also a good source of other essential vitamins. So, a handful of peanuts a day not only fulfills your biotin requirement but also the need for other vitamins that promote your overall health and keep you energetic throughout the day. The good fats present in peanuts add shine and luster to your hair and protect you from chronic diseases.

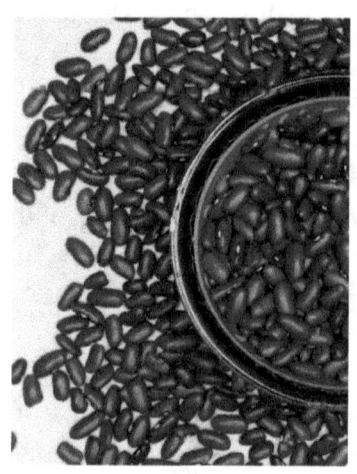

6. Kidney Beans

Kidney beans are rich in biotin. Half a cup of cooked kidney beans fulfills 17% of the daily requirement of vitamin H. They are not only a good source of biotin but also rich in protein, fibre, vitamin B9, vitamin K1 and essential minerals like copper, iron and potassium. Eating kidney beans with rice gives you a complete protein, which means this combination provides all the nine important amino acids that your body needs for proper functioning. They provide sustained energy and keep you full for a long time while aiding in weight management. They help keep your immune system functional. They promote digestive health, maintain normal blood sugar levels and protect your heart from diseases.

7. Sweet Potato

Sweet potato not only fulfills your biotin requirement, but it also has antioxidant and anti-inflammatory properties that successfully kill free radicals in your body and prevent inflammation and oxidative damage. This reduces the risk of developing diabetes, high blood pressure, cancer, and other serious diseases. It provides you with sustained energy and prevents sudden spikes in 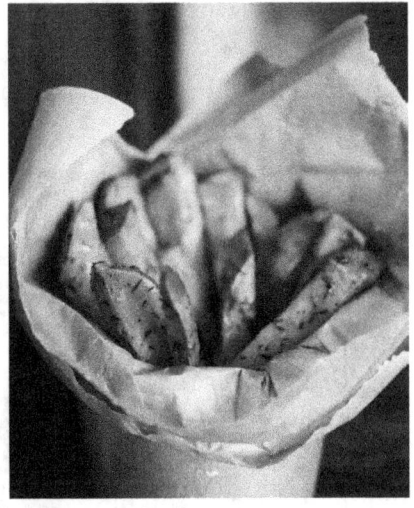 your blood sugar levels. One cooked sweet potato can fulfill 16% of your daily requirement of biotin.

8. Coffee

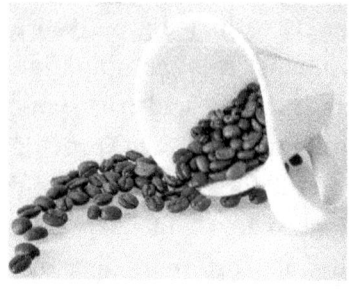

Coffee is a great source of vitamin B7. 100 grams of coffee contains 100 mcg of biotin. This means that a cup of coffee made from 1 tablespoon (about 6 grams) of instant coffee fulfills 20% of your daily requirement of biotin. Coffee is also good for your heart. It helps reduce the risk of diabetes, stroke, and cardiovascular diseases. It boosts energy by increasing the dopamine neurotransmitter in the brain and keeps you active and happy. However, coffee has a diuretic effect, which means it increases urination, and since B vitamins are water-soluble, excessive urination causes loss of these vitamins. So, consume coffee in moderation and eat foods rich in vitamin B after some time of drinking coffee.

9. Sunflower Seeds

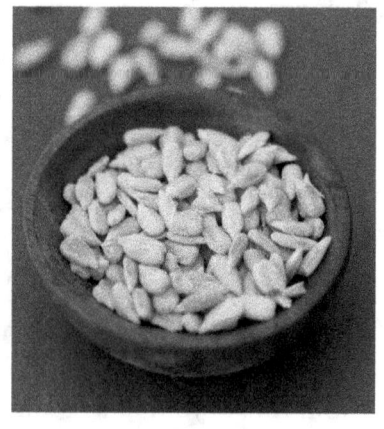

Sunflower seeds are a great way to add several water-soluble and fat-soluble vitamins to your body. Sunflower seeds contain a fair amount of biotin. A quarter cup of roasted sunflower seeds contains 2.6 mcg of biotin which is equal to 9% of the daily value of biotin.

The nutrients in sunflower seeds promote healthy skin, thicker hair, better immune function and prevention of cardiovascular diseases. Use sunflower seeds as a nut cream, add crushed seeds to your yogurt or eat them as is.

10. Strawberries

Strawberries are a good source of biotin and can fulfill your daily requirement of biotin. 100 grams of strawberries fulfill 5% of your body's daily requirement of biotin. Strawberries are high in antioxidants that help prevent oxidative damage by killing free radicals and thus prevent diseases caused by oxidative stress. They are low in calories and help in weight management. It helps lower blood pressure and prevents cardiovascular diseases. They are good for your skin, brain health and prevent various types of cancer.

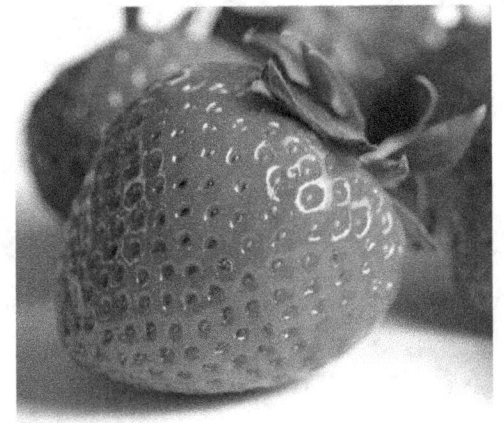

Other good sources of biotin are buckwheat, sorghum, milk, oats, bananas, flax seeds, beans, chickpeas, green peas, and avocado.

Chapter 7
VITAMIN B9

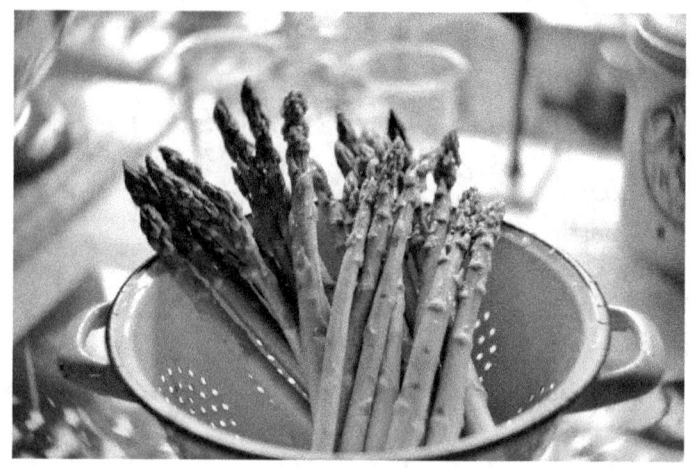

1.
EVERYTHING YOU NEED TO KNOW ABOUT VITAMIN B9

What is Vitamin B9, and what does it do?

The next essential water-soluble vitamin is Vitamin B9 which is also known as folate. Other names for folate are folacin, vitamin B11, vitamin BC, acidum folicum and folincyre. Folate is naturally present in vegetables, fruits, and beans as tetrahydrofolate (THF). Folate is required for DNA and RNA synthesis. It is also essential for the metabolism of amino acids. Folate exhibits its functions as a coenzyme, which is required by enzymes to carry out chemical reactions in the body.

What are the active forms of folate?

Folate cannot be absorbed as is, and it must be converted into its active form to perform its actions in the body. Only the active form of folate can cross the brain-blood-barrier (BBB). Folate is converted into its main biologically active form, 5-methyltetrahydrofolate (methylfolate or 5-MTHF), in the body.

Are folate and folic acid the same? If not, what is the difference between them?

Folate and folic acid are used interchangeably for vitamin B9. However, there is a difference between folate and folic acid. Folate is present in natural food, while folic acid is a man-made synthetic form of folate that is available as a supplement or added to fortified foods. Folic acid is also called monopteroylglutamic or pteroylmonoglutamic acid and is the oxidized form of vitamin B9. Most of the naturally occurring folates in food (about 90%) are polyglutamate, which means they contain more than one glutamate in their structure. On the other hand, folic acid is present as a monoglutamate, which means it contains only one glutamate.

Folate is highly sensitive and can be destroyed by heat, light, and oxidation. Folic acid is more stable than folate and cannot be destroyed by high temperatures, exposure to light, or oxidation.

All of the folate consumed is converted into its active form, 5-MTHF, in the digestive system, while some of the folic acid is converted into 5-MTHF in the liver.

How is vitamin B9 metabolized in the body?

The folate you consume through food has first to be absorbed into your body to perform any action. To be absorbed, folate must be converted into its active form. Naturally occurring folate in food is in the tetrahydrofolate (THF) form, which has more than one glutamate at its tail, making it a polyglutamate. The polyglutamate folate is converted into the monoglutamate form to be absorbed by active transport in your gut. The synthetic form of folate, i.e., folic acid, is absorbed through passive diffusion. The monoglutamate form is converted to dihydrofolate (DHF) before it enters your bloodstream, and dihydrofolate reductase converts it to tetrahydrofolate (THF). Enzymes then convert THF to the active form 5-methyltetrahydrofolate (5-MTHF).

Unmetabolized folic acid in the body is not uncommon. When dihydrofolate reductase capacity is exceeded, it cannot convert DHF to THF, and folic acid remains unmetabolized in your blood. Your body can process only a limited amount of folic acid at a time, and unmetabolized folic acid is excreted through urine. Some studies suggest that unmetabolized folic acid is linked to certain health problems, although no health risks or health benefits from unmetabolized folic acid have yet been established.

Is vitamin B9 stored in the body?

Vitamin B9 is water-soluble, so it dissolves in water and is easily excreted through urine. Your body does not store vitamin B9 for long periods, so you need to get it through food every day. Your body typically stores folate for up to 4 months. However, your body does not store large amounts of folate; the total stored content of folate is about 15 to 30 mg, with about half stored in the liver and the rest in the blood and body tissues.

Since folate is not stored well in large amounts, a deficiency can occur within a few weeks to months of eating a folate-deficient diet.

Is vitamin B9 really an essential nutrient?

Although vitamin B9 is essential and must be taken through food, your body can also make some folate and contribute to its status. Your colonic microbiota synthesizes some folate and can be absorbed in the colon. However, how much colonic folate contributes to folate status in the body is not yet known. Therefore, until we know more about the contribution of colonic folate, folate will remain an essential water-soluble vitamin that you must consume through food every day for normal bodily functions.

How much vitamin B9 do I need a day?

Folate is naturally present in food; however, its bioavailability is poor compared to the synthetic oxidized form, folic acid, which is taken as a supplement or added to foods that do not naturally contain this vitamin to avoid folate deficiency. Bioavailability refers to the actual amount of the active form of a vitamin that reaches your blood circulation and exerts its action. The structure of folate and folic acid plays a major role in the bioavailability of this vitamin. Folate contains more glutamates (polyglutamate), while folic acid contains only one glutamate (monoglutamate). Therefore, folate undergoes one more step, i.e., it is first broken down into monoglutamate while folic acid is already in the monoglutamate form, so it is readily available to be converted into the active form. The bioavailability of folate naturally present in food is 50%, while the bioavailability of folic acid when taken with food is 85%. Therefore, the current RDA for folate is expressed as mcg of dietary folate equivalents (DFE). The officially defined DFE is as follows:

1 mcg DFE = 1 mcg food folate
1 mcg DFE = 0.5 mcg folic acid (vitamin supplement taken on an empty stomach)
1 mcg DFE = 0.6 mcg folic acid (present in fortified foods or vitamin supplements when consumed with foods)

The daily average recommended level of vitamin B9 intake that is sufficient to meet your body's requirement is given below:

Age	Male	Female
Birth to 6 m*	65 mcg DFE*	65 mcg DFE*
7–12 m*	80 mcg DFE*	80 mcg DFE*
1–3 yrs.	150 mcg DFE	150 mcg DFE
4–8 yrs.	200 mcg DFE	200 mcg DFE
9–13 yrs.	300 mcg DFE	300 mcg DFE
14+ yrs.	400 mcg DFE	400 mcg DFE

*Adequate Intake (AI): Assumed level to ensure nutritional adequacy.

What factors can be responsible for folate deficiency?

Folate deficiency is common, except in countries where folic acid fortification programs are in place. Below are some of the common causes of folate deficiency:

Poor diet: A poor diet that lacks folate-rich foods such as raw green vegetables and whole grains can lead to low folate levels in your body.

Prolonged cooking: Folate is heat sensitive. Cooking natural folate-rich foods for a long time destroys their folate content. So, even if you are eating a high folate-rich diet, if they are cooked for a long time, it can result in folate deficiency.

Alcoholism: People who have a chronic drinking habit usually replace nutritious food with alcohol, which can lead to a deficiency of vitamin B9. Alcohol also interferes with folate absorption, metabolism, and excretion, contributing to its deficiency.

Certain medical conditions: People on kidney dialysis are at risk of folate deficiency. Dialysis increases urinary excretion, and as vitamin B9 is water-soluble, it is quickly excreted without being absorbed by the body.

Pregnancy and nursing: Pregnancy and nursing increase the body's demand for folic acid, which, if not met, can lead to a deficiency of this vitamin.

Malabsorption: Any vitamin must first be properly absorbed to provide health benefits. Certain diseases, like celiac disease, and the use of certain medications, like antiseizure drugs, can impede the absorption of folate in the body. The active form of folate cannot reach your blood circulation to perform its action without being properly absorbed, resulting in folate deficiency.

Folate antagonists: Certain medications like the drug used in diabetes, metformin, anti-rheumatic medicines such as methotrexate, antibiotics-trimethoprim and sulfamethoxazole, anti-hypertensive medication: triamterene and antiseizure medications, interfere with the metabolism of folate and do not allow it to be converted into its active form in your body. Folate cannot perform its essential function without being converted into its active form. This leads to folate deficiency.

Does cooking and exposure to light destroy the folate in my food?

Folate is susceptible to deterioration due to heat and sunlight. Cooking folate-rich food for a long duration can destroy up to 40% of the folate present in them. Baking can destroy up to 70% of the folate of the food. The process of milling grains to make flour also generates heat that can destroy up to 70% of their folate content.

Spending more time in sunlight is good for increasing your vitamin D levels; however, it can affect your body's folate status. Folate is sensitive to sunlight. The ultraviolet (UV) radiation of the sun can degrade folate, especially in pregnant women. Folic acid is usually prescribed during pregnancy to deal with any folate deficiency and protect the baby's health.

What happens if I consume too much folate?

Taking folate from natural sources does not cause any major adverse effects; however, this is not true when you meet your body's folate requirement through folic acid supplements. Excess folic acid is usually excreted through urine. However, taking high doses of folic acid over a long period can hide vitamin B12 deficiency (if you have it) until the neurological side effects become irreversible. This is why folic acid and vitamin B12 are usually prescribed together. Other side effects of excess folic acid include nausea, diarrhea, stomach pain, irritation, skin reactions, confusion, and slow brain development in children.

What if I am deficient in vitamin B9?

Vitamin B9 is essential for DNA synthesis, energy production, and proper growth and development. Folate deficiency can lead to the following diseases:

Megaloblastic anemia: Folate deficiency can cause a specific type of anemia called megaloblastic anemia. Folate is involved in DNA synthesis and cell division, which is essential for your body's normal development and growth. Folate deficiency disrupts DNA synthesis, which prevents nuclear division. This leads to the formation of larger-than-normal red blood cells that affect the oxygen-carrying capacity of RBCs and can cause symptoms of shortness of breath, fatigue, and weakness.

Megaloblastic anemia can also occur due to vitamin B12 deficiency, so diagnostic tests are needed to determine whether it is caused by folate or vitamin B12 deficiency.

Neural tube birth defects in babies: Folate is important for the development of the central nervous system. Vitamin B9 deficiency in pregnant women can cause birth defects called neural tube defects (NTDs), including spina bifida, in the developing fetus. Folic acid also reduces the chances of miscarriage. Therefore, women who are pregnant or planning to get pregnant should consult their doctor for the proper dosage of folic acid supplements.

Cardiovascular diseases: Vitamin B9, along with vitamins B6 and B12, is involved in regulating homocysteine levels in your blood. High homocysteine concentrations in the body are associated with an increased risk of heart disease as it is involved in damaging blood vessels and promoting blood clots.

Folate is needed to break down homocysteine into other chemical compounds essential for your body. Folate is required for the remethylation of homocysteine into the essential amino acid, methionine, which lowers homocysteine levels.

Cancer: Folate deficiency may increase your risk of cancer. Folate plays an irreplaceable role in DNA synthesis, cell division, and methylation. DNA damage, impaired DNA repair, and improper gene expression are the major causes of cancer. Folate deficiency affects DNA synthesis and repair, which may lead to genome instability and chromosome breakage, leading to cancer development.

What are the symptoms of folate deficiency?

A person with vitamin B9 deficiency may have the following symptoms:

- Mouth ulcers
- Gray hair
- Weakness, fatigue
- Decreased appetite
- Glossitis (Swollen tongue)
- Shortness of breath
- Poor growth
- Forgetfulness

How is vitamin B9 deficiency diagnosed?

RBC and Serum Folate Concentrations: Red blood cell and serum folate concentrations are commonly used to determine folate status. Serum folate indicates recent dietary intake, such as how much folate has been circulating in the blood in the last few hours, and does not reflect long-term status.

Since the RBC folate test is derived from red blood cells, it provides a long-term measure of folate intake, i.e., how much folate a person has taken in recent weeks.

The healthy range for serum folate concentrations:

Greater than 3 ng/mL indicates adequate folate levels.

The healthy range for RBC folate concentrations:

Greater than 140 ng/mL indicates adequate folate levels.

Plasma Homocysteine Concentration: This is commonly used as a functional indicator of folate status. Homocysteine levels increase in your blood when your body cannot convert homocysteine to methionine due to a deficiency of the folate active form 5-MTHF.

The test ranges are given below:
10 micromol/L and lower: Normal
12 to 14 micromol/L: Borderline
16 micromol/L: Elevated homocysteine level

This method is not a specific indicator of folate status because homocysteine levels can be affected by other conditions such as vitamin B12 deficiency, vitamin B6 deficiency, and kidney dysfunction.

2. IMPORTANCE OF VITAMIN B9

Folate has many important functions in your body. Folate exerts its action through its active forms that act as cofactors for enzymes responsible for carrying out various chemical reactions in your body. Some of the most critical functions of folate are given below:

FUNCTIONS OF FOLATE IN THE BODY

Synthesis of Nucleic Acids

Folate helps your body make new cells. Folate is involved in synthesizing nucleic acids (DNA and RNA) as well as cell replication and growth. Folate coenzymes are needed in the synthesis of DNA from thymidine and purines. It is also necessary to convert homocysteine to methionine, which is required to synthesize S-adenosylmethionine (SAM). SAM is essential in methylation within DNA, RNA, and proteins. DNA methylation is an important function that regulates gene expression and is necessary for assigning specific structures and functions to the cells that enable them to perform a certain task in your body. Any defect in DNA methylation is associated with the development of cancer.

Metabolism of Amino Acids

The active forms of folate act as coenzymes and participate in the metabolism of several important amino acids, including methionine, histidine, cysteine, serine, and glycine. Your body breaks down these amino acids into important chemicals that are used in many reactions necessary for the normal functioning of your body.

Red Blood Cell Formation

Folate is required for DNA synthesis and cell division, which is necessary for the normal development and growth of your body not only in childhood but throughout your life. It prevents DNA mutations. Proper methylation, DNA synthesis, and nuclear division are required for the normal and healthy maturation of red blood cells. Folate is responsible for the methylation of deoxyuridylate to thymidylate in DNA formation, which is essential for proper cell division. Any impairment in this reaction inhibits cell division, which negatively affects the maturation of RBCs, resulting in irregular and larger-than-normal RBCs. These abnormal RBCs die quickly and have a reduced capacity to carry oxygen. This reduces the blood supply to your body tissues, leading to fatigue and weakness.

Maintain Homocysteine Levels

The most important role of folate is to convert homocysteine to methionine. Homocysteine is metabolized by two pathways: remethylation to methionine, which depends on folate and vitamin B12, and transsulfuration to cystathionine, which requires vitamin B6. Methylation of homocysteine to methionine is facilitated by 5-methyl-tetrahydrofolate (5-MTHF), a form of folate. This conversion is catalyzed by the methionine synthase enzyme, which requires vitamin B12 as a cofactor to produce its action. Without enough folate in your body, this remethylation cannot occur, which raises homocysteine levels and increases your risk of heart attack and stroke.

Happy Hormones Production

The active forms of folate are involved in the synthesis of essential neurotransmitters in the brain, such as norepinephrine, serotonin, and dopamine. These neurotransmitters act as hormones and control how you feel and sleep. Dopamine is responsible for your excitement. It helps you feel pleasure and rewards. It helps you focus and keeps you motivated. While dopamine is responsible for sudden excitement and happiness, serotonin is responsible for well-being, long-lasting happiness, and calmness. Serotonin aids in digestion and helps regulate your sleep-wake cycle. Norepinephrine plays an essential role in increasing alertness, arousal, attention, mood, cognitive activities, and stress responses.

Antioxidant and Anti-Inflammatory Properties

Several studies suggest that folate, in its active form, has free radical scavenging properties and prevents lipid peroxidation. Folate indirectly prevents oxidative stress by reducing homocysteine concentrations, which helps increase the body's antioxidant capacity and reduce free radical formation.

Inflammation is the leading cause of many chronic diseases. Folate may help reduce inflammation in your body. It reduces the concentrations of inflammatory markers such as C-reactive protein (CRP) in your body, an inflammatory protein that increases when there is inflammation in your body.

TOP HEALTH BENEFITS OF VITAMIN B9

1. Mouth Ulcers: Getting enough folate through natural sources can help you prevent mouth ulcers. Folic acid can reduce the occurrence, intensity, and duration of mouth ulcers. It facilitates the healing process of the oral mucosa, reduces inflammation, and heals ulcers quickly. Not just mouth ulcers, vitamin B9 also has beneficial effects on other oral health problems like periodontitis and gingivitis, which, if left untreated, can lead to tooth loss and other health issues. Several studies suggest that vitamin B9 helps manage these conditions by promoting gum health and reducing inflammation.

2. Regulate the Menstrual Cycle: Regular and adequate folate intake helps regulate your menstrual cycle. Folate regulates the regularity of your menstrual cycle, the duration of menstruation, and the intensity of menstrual flow. Folate is essential for hormonal balance; it increases progesterone levels. Low levels of vitamin B9 can affect the way your body deals with the hormone estrogen, resulting in hormonal imbalance, which is the major cause of heavy menstrual periods, polycystic ovary syndrome (PCOS), and fibroids. In addition, folate helps your ovaries function better by reducing the amino acid homocysteine levels in the ovaries, and this can lengthen your menstrual cycle. Folic acid also helps prevent anemia associated with heavy menstrual periods.

3. Promote A Healthy Pregnancy: It is especially important to consume adequate amounts of folate during pregnancy. Folate promotes a healthy pregnancy and prevents various adverse pregnancy outcomes. It also reduces the chances of miscarriage. Folate is essential for the early development of the fetus. It helps prevent neural tube defects, cardiac abnormalities, and orofacial clefts in the baby. Taking adequate amounts of folate during pregnancy helps reduce the risk of autism spectrum disorder in the baby. This is why folic acid supplements are prescribed during pregnancy.

4. Protect Cardiovascular Health: Elevated homocysteine levels increase your risk of atherosclerosis. High levels of Homocysteine damage the blood vessels and hamper smooth, unrestricted blood flow to your heart. It promotes clotting in the blood vessels, which causes cardiovascular diseases. Folate, along with vitamins B12 and B6, helps reduce homocysteine levels by breaking it down into other essential chemicals. High folate intake ensures low homocysteine levels and protects your heart from various disorders.

5. Natural Antidepressant and Prevents Neurodegenerative Disorders: High intake of folate through fruits and vegetables is associated with a lower risk of depression, memory loss, dementia, and Alzheimer's disease. Vitamin B9 promotes brain health in various ways. Folate is involved in the synthesis of various neurotransmitters, like serotonin, norepinephrine, and dopamine, that help improve your mood and prevent depression. These neurotransmitters are found deficient in depression. Folate prevents and treats depression by promoting the synthesis of antidepressant neurotransmitters in your brain.

Folate prevents brain diseases such as dementia, memory loss, Alzheimer's, and stroke. It plays an important role in nucleic acid (DNA and RNA) synthesis and methylation reactions, which are important for normal brain development and function. Additionally, folate helps reduce homocysteine levels and increase healthy red blood cell production, which enhances brain function and prevents strokes associated with blood clots caused by high homocysteine levels.

6. Prevent Cancer: Folate reduces your risk of certain types of cancer, including breast cancer, cervical, colon, pancreatic, and stomach cancer. Folate is essential in the synthesis of DNA, RNA, and proteins; it helps in the methylation of DNA and promotes cell division. The antioxidant property of folate helps prevent oxidative damage to DNA. Any defect in DNA makes you vulnerable to cancer. Folate helps prevent the mutation of DNA, which is one of many causes of cancer. While healthy folate levels in your body are linked to a lower risk of various types of cancer, high doses of folic acid through supplements, have also been associated with an increased risk of prostate cancer.

7. Prevent Anemia: Vitamin B9 helps prevent and treat megaloblastic anemia. Poor and low red blood cell production in your body leads to anemia. Due to anemia, your blood does not have enough healthy RBCs to carry oxygen and nutrients to all your tissues and organs, and you feel weak and tired. Folate aids in the production of red blood cells. It aids in the maturation of young red blood cells and promotes healthy RBC production.

8. Increases Women's Fertility: Folate is a must for pregnant women or women trying to conceive. A folate-rich diet increases your chances of getting pregnant and supports a healthy pregnancy. Folate plays an important role in improving egg quality. It aids in synthesizing the egg's DNA molecule, promotes egg growth, and helps them implant in the uterus. Taking folate can increase your chances of getting pregnant and carrying a baby to term.

3.
10 RICHEST VEGETARIAN SOURCES OF VITAMIN B9

Below are the 10 richest vegetarian food sources of Vitamin B9 (Folate):

1. Dark Green Leafy Vegetable

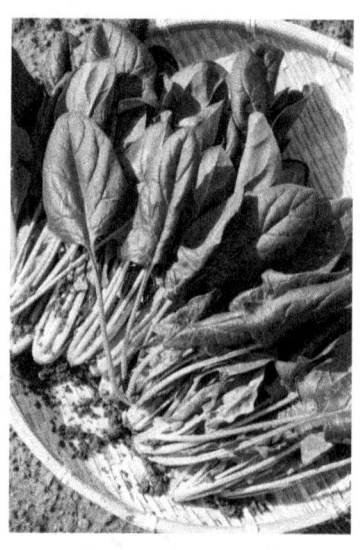

Dark green leafy vegetables are an excellent source of vitamin B9. They are also rich in other essential nutrients that provide you with sustained energy and promote your overall health. Half a cup of cooked spinach fulfills 33% of your body's daily requirement of vitamin B9. While half a cup of boiled mustard greens fulfills 13%

of the daily value of folate. Dark green leafy vegetables protect you from cancer to a great extent as they have high antioxidant content. They have anti-inflammatory properties and they protect you from inflammatory diseases like arthritis by reducing inflammation in your body. In fact, they can protect your bones from osteoporosis as they are high in vitamin K.

2. Cowpeas

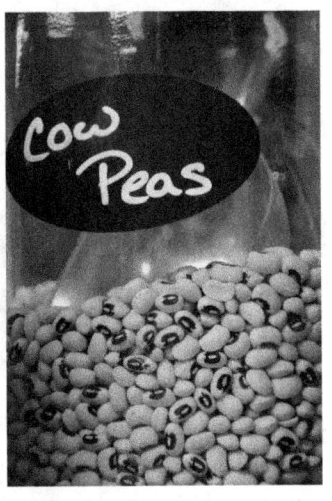

Cowpeas or black eye peas are an excellent source of vitamin B9. Half a cup of cooked cowpeas contains 26% of the daily value of folate. Cowpeas are rich in protein, fibre, other vitamins and flavonoids. The high content of flavonoids, potassium, magnesium and folate in cowpeas improves your heart functioning and protects your heart health. They help lower cholesterol levels in your body as they are rich in cholesterol-lowering phytosterols. They increase the production of red blood cells and ensure that all your organs receive oxygen and nutrient-rich blood so that they can work efficiently.

3. Asparagus

Asparagus is rich in folate. Four spears of cooked asparagus fulfill 22% of your body's requirement of folate. The high vitamin K content in them helps promote your bone health. They are high in antioxidants like vitamin E and glutathione that help your body fight free radicals and reduce their cell-damaging effects. They strengthen your immune system and are low in calories and rich in fiber and water which aids in weight management.

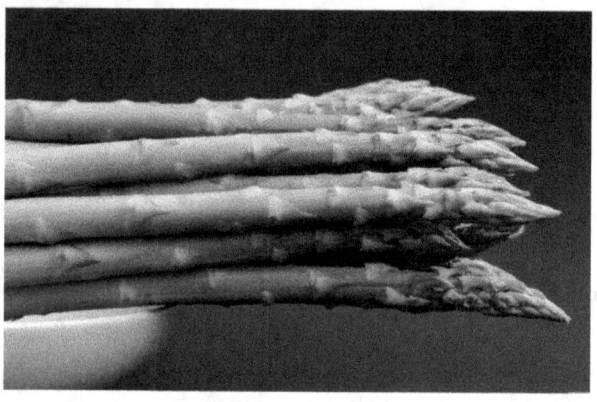

Asparagus is a natural diuretic, it increases urine production and helps treat urinary tract infections. However, being a diuretic it flushes out water-soluble vitamins from your body faster. So, eat foods rich in vitamin B and C some time after munching on asparagus.

4. Cruciferous Vegetable Family

Members of the cruciferous vegetable family like Brussels sprouts, broccoli, cabbage and cauliflower are excellent sources of folate. Cruciferous vegetables are known to protect against cancer. They are rich in vitamin A, C and vitamin B9. They are high in omega-

3 fats which are known to reduce inflammation in the body. These healthy fats promote cognitive health, reducing the risk of memory loss, mental decline, and Alzheimer's disease. 1 cup of cooked Brussels

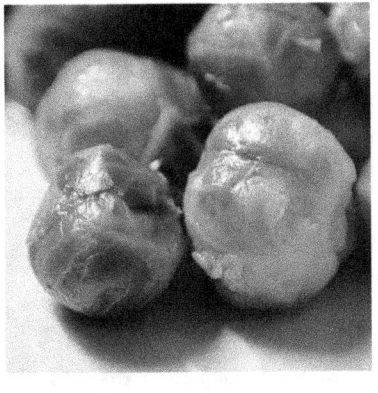

sprouts meets 40% daily requirement of folate, 1 cup of cooked broccoli 26%, 1 cup of cooked cauliflower 14% and 1 cup of cooked cabbage meets 12% daily requirement of vitamin B9.

5. Avocado

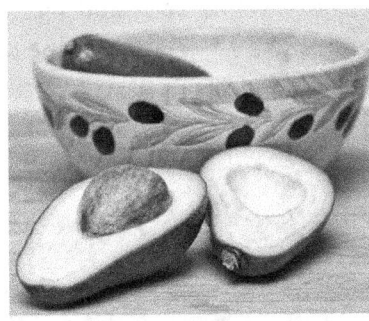

Avocados are a delicious way to increase your vitamin and healthy fat consumption. They are packed with folate. 1 medium avocado can fulfill 22% of your body's daily requirement of folate. They are also rich in other B vitamins that increase your energy levels and help your body function efficiently. They keep your brain healthy and aid in healthy growth and development. They promote natural detoxification and the healthy fats in avocados protect you from serious diseases and promote overall health.

6. Kidney Beans and Soybeans

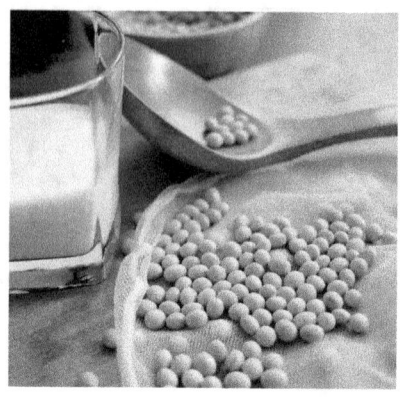

Beans like kidney beans and soybeans are a great source of vitamin B9. They are also packed with other B vitamins, protein, and fiber. They are good for digestion and provide you with energy throughout the day. Beans aid in the production of healthy red blood cells and prevent birth defects such as neural tube defects in the developing fetus. Half a cup of cooked kidney beans fulfills 29% of the folate required in a day, half a cup of cooked soybeans fulfills 12%, and half a cup of cooked green soybeans has a 25% daily value of folate.

7. Beetroot

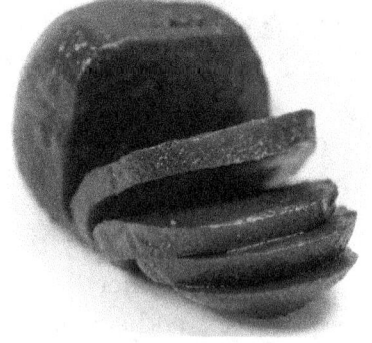

Beetroot is rich in nutrients. They are rich in folate, potassium, iron, manganese, and vitamin C. They are high in nitrates, which cause vasodilation and keep your blood pressure normal. They protect heart health and increase stamina. The high antioxidants present in beetroot help kill free radicals and prevent cell-damaging oxidative stress. One beetroot can fulfill 23% of your body's daily folate requirement.

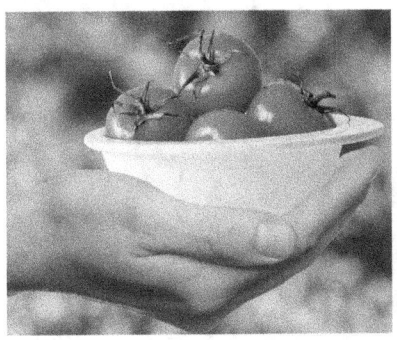

8. Tomatoes

Tomatoes are a great source of folate. One large tomato (180 grams) contains 7% of the daily value of folate. They are also a great source of vitamin C, K, and potassium. Lycopene is a potent antioxidant responsible for tomatoes' red color and is associated with countless health benefits, including a reduced risk of cancer, hypertension, and cardiovascular disease. Another plant compound in tomatoes, naringenin, is a flavonoid that reduces inflammation and protects against various chronic diseases.

9. Citrus Fruits

Citrus fruits like oranges, lemons, and grapefruits are good sources of folate. Even though they may not meet 100% of your daily folate requirement, they can certainly meet some of your folate requirements in a day. One orange contains 14% of the daily value of folate, while half a grapefruit contains 4% of your daily recommended folate. Citrus fruits are essentially rich in vitamin C, which helps boost your immunity, protect you from infections, and keep your skin fresh and moist.

10. Sweet Corn

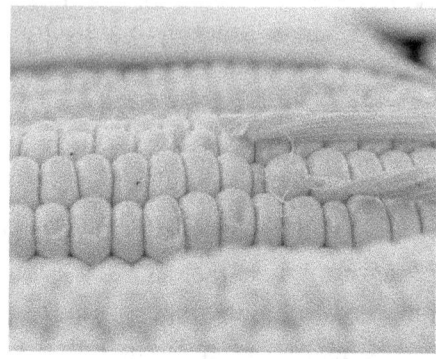

Sweet corns are a good source of folate. One 7' long sweet corn contains 15% of the daily requirement of folate. They are high in dietary fiber, which keeps you full for longer and prevents food cravings. Fibre aids digestion and helps reduce the risk of bowel cancer, diabetes, heart disorders and stroke. They are also rich in vitamins B3, B5, B6 and potassium. They are packed with antioxidants that protect your eyes from oxidative damage and boost eye health.

Other good sources of folate are sunflower seeds (a quarter cup contains 21% DV), peanuts (a quarter cup contains 22% DV), flax seeds (a tablespoon contains 7% DV), papaya (one small fruit contains 15% DV), okra or ladyfinger (one cup cooked contains 10% DV), and wheat germ (1 tablespoon contains 5% DV). This variety of sources offers an exciting opportunity to explore new foods and flavors while reaping the health benefits of folate.

Chapter 8
VITAMIN B12

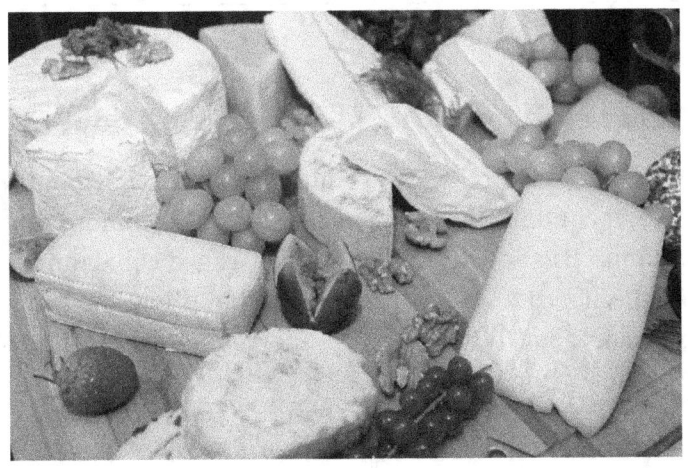

1.
EVERYTHING YOU NEED TO KNOW ABOUT VITAMIN B12

What is vitamin B12, and what does it do?

Our last essential water-soluble B vitamin is vitamin B12. It contains the cobalt mineral, so compounds with vitamin B12 activity are collectively called cobalamins. Vitamin B12 is needed for the function and development of the central nervous system, DNA synthesis, and normal red blood cell formation.

What are the active forms of vitamin B12?

Vitamin B12 itself is not active and cannot be absorbed without being converted into active forms. In your body, vitamin B12 is converted into its biologically active forms, methylcobalamin and 5-deoxyadenosylcobalamin. The active forms of vitamin B12 act as a cofactor for two important enzymes, methionine synthase and L-methylmalonyl-CoA mutase. These enzymes cannot perform their actions in your body without vitamin B12. The other two forms that can be converted into the primary active forms of vitamin B12 are hydroxycobalamin and cyanocobalamin.

Natural food sources contain vitamin B12 in the form of methylcobalamin. Methylcobalamin is also used in dietary supplements. Cyanocobalamin is a man-made synthetic form of vitamin B12 that is not available in nature. It is generally used as a vitamin supplement or in fortified foods. It can be converted into the active forms of vitamin B12 i.e. methylcobalamin or adenosylcobalamin.

How is vitamin B12 metabolized in the body?

Vitamin B12 is bound to proteins in your vitamin B12-containing food. It must first be freed to be absorbed. This process begins when food mixes with saliva in your mouth, which frees some of the vitamin B12 from the protein complex. These protein-free vitamin B12 bind to another cobalamin-binding protein called haptocorrin in your saliva. The rest of the protein-bound vitamin B12 from your food is freed by hydrochloric acid and gastric proteases in the stomach, which then bind to haptocorrin. Digestive enzymes break down the vitamin B12-haptocorrin complex in the duodenum (part of the small intestine), and the free vitamin B12 forms a complex with a transport and delivery binding protein called intrinsic factor. Vitamin B12 is then absorbed in the last part of the small intestine, the ileum. Fortified foods or dietary supplements contain free vitamin B12, so they do not need to be separated.

Is vitamin B12 stored in the body?

Unlike fat-soluble vitamins, vitamin B12 is not stored in your body. It dissolves in water, and excess amounts are excreted through urine. However, the body stores some amount of vitamin B12 in the liver. Your body stores about 1 mg to 5 mg of vitamin B12, about 1000 to 2000 times more than the average amount consumed daily, which can last for about 2 to 5 years. Therefore, there may be cases where symptoms of vitamin B12 deficiency may not develop even after years, but you may still have vitamin B12 deficiency.

Is vitamin B12 really an essential nutrient?

Although vitamin B12 is an essential vitamin and must be taken in through food, your body can also make vitamin B12, which can contribute greatly to its status. Certain bacteria present in your gut can synthesize vitamin B12. Your gut bacteria can produce as well as require vitamin B12 for metabolic reactions. About 20% of gut bacteria can synthesize vitamin B12, but more than 80% of gut bacteria require B12 for their metabolic reactions. Two common species, Lactobacillus and Bifidobacterium, can produce vitamin B12 in the gut. The gut flora in humans is highly diverse. Therefore, the synthesis capacity of vitamin B12 also varies from person to person. Additionally, a person's intake of vitamin B12-rich food also affects the synthesis of this vitamin. This is why even though the body can make vitamin B12, it is still considered an essential vitamin, and you must get it through food sources.

How much vitamin B12 do I need a day?

The amount of vitamin B12 intake required to maintain healthy serum vitamin B12 levels for healthy individuals is given below:

Age	Male	Female
Birth to 6 m*	0.4 mcg	0.4 mcg
7–12 m*	0.5 mcg	0.5 mcg
1–3 yrs.	0.9 mcg	0.9 mcg
4–8 yrs.	1.2 mcg	1.2 mcg
9–13 yrs.	1.8 mcg	1.8 mcg
14+ yrs.	2.4 mcg	2.4 mcg

* Adequate Intake (AI)

What factors can lead to vitamin B12 deficiency?

The following factors can be responsible for vitamin B12 deficiency:

Inadequate intake: Vitamin B12 is present in animal sources, and people who follow restricted diets, like veganism and fad, can suffer from vitamin B12 deficiency. If a nursing mother follows a restricted diet, her baby is at risk of developing vitamin B12 deficiency.

Aging: As you age, your stomach acidity decreases. Vitamin B12 in food is bound to proteins that need to be freed. Stomach acidity is needed to release vitamin B12 from the vitamin B12-protein complex. When stomach acidity is low your body's absorption of vitamin B12 is reduced and you do not get the benefits of this vitamin. Vitamin B12 found in vitamin supplements is in free form which can be absorbed well even in people with reduced stomach acid.

Liver disorders: Most vitamin B12 is stored in your liver. Liver disorders affect vitamin B12 storage, reducing vitamin B12 levels in your body and leading to vitamin B12 deficiency.

Infections: Infections like fish tapeworm infection and blind loop syndrome can cause vitamin B12 deficiency. Fish tapeworm infection occurs when you eat raw or undercooked meat contaminated with fish tapeworm larvae that grow in your intestine. Similarly, blind loop syndrome occurs due to excessive growth of bacteria in your intestine. These bacteria compete for vitamin B12 in your body and force vitamin B12 to pass to them. They absorb vitamin B12 from the food the infected person consumes, which can lead to vitamin B12 deficiency and megaloblastic anemia.

Certain disease conditions

Inflammatory bowel disease: This condition affects the last section of your small intestine where vitamin B12 is absorbed resulting in low levels of vitamin B12 in your body.

Malabsorption disorders: Certain disease conditions like celiac disease and pancreatic disorders impair the absorption of vitamin B12 in the body resulting in inadequate levels of this vitamin.

Pernicious anemia: Pernicious anemia causes vitamin B12 deficiency. It is an autoimmune disease that prevents the absorption of vitamin B12 in your body. Intrinsic factor is a protein manufactured in your stomach that helps absorb vitamin B12. Intrinsic factor is not produced in pernicious anemia. As a result, people with pernicious anemia cannot absorb vitamin B12 from food despite taking a vitamin B12-rich diet.

Metaplastic atrophic gastritis: It is an autoimmune disease in which intrinsic factor is deficient. The overactive immune system produces abnormal antibodies that attack and destroy intrinsic factor-producing stomach cells, preventing the absorption of vitamin B12 ingested through food.

Certain medications

Antacids: If you are taking medications (antacids) to reduce acidity which are also prescribed with antibiotics then your vitamin B12 levels may be low. Antacids reduce stomach acidity required to release vitamin B12 from the vitamin B12-protein complex of food. Without enough stomach acid, your body cannot absorb vitamin B12 even if you are consuming enough vitamin B12-rich foods.

Antidiabetic medication: Metformin is the first-line drug prescribed for treating diabetes. It interferes with the metabolism of vitamin B12 and can make you vitamin B12 deficient.

Nitrous Oxide (Laughing Gas): Repeated exposure to laughing gas, nitrous oxide, can make you vitamin B12 deficient. Nitrous oxide is commonly used in anesthesia, it destroys methylcobalamin, leading to vitamin B12 deficiency.

Surgery: Some conditions require the removal of a part of the stomach. Bariatric surgery also involves removing a portion of the stomach for weight loss. When the intrinsic factor producing part of the stomach is surgically removed, it prevents the absorption of vitamin B12 in the body and results in vitamin B12 deficiency.

Does cooking, light exposure, and alkali destroy vitamin B12 in my food?

Vitamin B12 is not heat sensitive, which means cooking does not reduce the amount of vitamin B12 in food. However, vitamin B12 is sensitive to light and alkali. Just like folate, vitamin B12 is destroyed by exposure to sunlight. Solar radiation can destroy vitamin B12 in your skin.

Vitamin B12 is destroyed by alkali solutions. Therefore, using baking soda with food containing vitamin B12 can destroy B12 in your food. If you are taking antacids for indigestion and acidity, it can also destroy vitamin B12 and reduce its levels in your body. Even your toothpaste can destroy vitamin B12.

Is RO-processed drinking water lowering my vitamin B12 levels?

Let's first understand RO and TDS:

Total Dissolved Solids (TDS): All substances dissolved in water other than H2O, including organic and inorganic elements such as minerals, salts, metals, and ions, are classified as Total Dissolved Solids (TDS).

Reverse Osmosis (RO): Reverse Osmosis (RO) is a process of purifying water by removing salt or water hardness and other heavy metals and unwanted molecules from drinking water. Reverse osmosis uses a partially permeable membrane to filter out unwanted molecules.

Water contains naturally dissolved essential minerals, including calcium, magnesium, and cobalt. It may also contain harmful heavy metals like lead. The purpose of purifying water through RO is to remove non-water substances from water. However, extensive RO filtration can reduce TDS to below-standard levels. Extensive removal by RO removes healthy dissolved minerals, including cobalt, from water, which can be harmful to your health. Cobalt is an important part of vitamin B12 composition. Low-mineralized water reduces the absorption of vitamin B12 in your body. Without being well absorbed, vitamin B12 cannot perform its function. As we have discussed above, vitamin B12 can be produced by gut flora; these require cobalt to synthesize vitamin B12.

Studies have confirmed that extensive RO filtration contributes to reduced vitamin B12 levels in the human body. However, large-scale studies are needed to determine the TDS levels that affect vitamin B12 as these studies have not been conducted on a large group of people, and the actual TDS levels of the RO-purified water used in the studies have not been specified. Hence, it is not yet clear how low TDS affects vitamin B12 levels in the body. Lower than normal TDS may affect vitamin B12 levels in your body, but water with the official healthy TDS level is suitable for drinking.

The TDS level for normal fresh water (not RO-processed water) is given below:

TDS in Water (measured in PPM)	Suitability for Drinking
Between 50-150	Excellent
150-250	Good, in terms of cardiovascular health
250-300	Fair
300-500	Not great: Consider an RO system to filter TDS
900-1200	Poor, not fit for drinking
Above 1200	Not acceptable

A TDS level of 50-150 is ideal for drinking natural fresh water, as it contains natural minerals. However, if you are drinking RO-purified water, the TDS level in the purified water should not be less than 80 ppm. At less than 80 ppm, the dissolved minerals are removed along with heavy metals. Some water purifiers add minerals such as calcium and magnesium, but they are not as effective as natural freshwater because the RO system removes many other micronutrients dissolved in water that benefit your health.

Keep a TDS meter at your home, which is readily available in the market. Check the TDS of your water supply. If the hardness of your water supply is more than 300 ppm, then only use an RO system; otherwise, use a UV filter to clean your drinking water. If you are using an RO system, check the TDS of your purified water, and if it is less than 80 ppm, ask your water purifier service provider to adjust the TDS level in the system.

What happens if I consume too much vitamin B12?

High intakes of vitamin B12 through foods and supplements are not associated with any adverse health effects. Since the body does not store excess vitamin B12, large amounts of vitamin B12 are generally considered safe. However, too much of anything may not be good for health, especially if it comes from supplements.

What happens if I am deficient in vitamin B12?

Megaloblastic anemia: Your body needs vitamin B12 to produce healthy red blood cells. Without enough vitamin B12, your body cannot produce healthy red blood cells, leading to larger-than-normal red blood cell production with reduced oxygen-carrying capacity, known as megaloblastic anemia.

Birth defects in the baby: Vitamin B12 deficiency in pregnant women and nursing mothers can cause neural tube defects, developmental delays, and anemia in the offspring.

Depression: Vitamin B12 deficiency plays a crucial role in generating depressive symptoms. Vitamin B12 deficiency increases homocysteine levels and oxidative stress while reducing energy production, which all cumulatively impairs neurotransmitter signals and causes the death of nerve cells, which initiates depression.

Infertility in Men: Vitamin B12 deficiency can lead to infertility, the inability to conceive in men. Vitamin B12 plays a key role in the formation, maturation, and movement of sperm. Vitamin B12 deficiency affects sperm count and can cause temporary infertility.

Dementia and cognitive impairment: Vitamin B12 plays a vital role in reducing the homocysteine levels in your body. Increased levels of homocysteine are directly linked to the incidence of Alzheimer's disease and dementia. Vitamin B12 deficiency increases homocysteine levels, which can damage the blood vessels in your brain and restrict blood flow to the brain. This deprives the brain of essential energy and nutrients and results in dementia, Alzheimer's disease, and other neurodegenerative diseases.

Cardiovascular diseases: Elevated levels of homocysteine can damage arteries and prevent the smooth flow of blood to your heart, increasing the risk of cardiovascular diseases. Vitamin B12, along with other B vitamins, is involved in the breakdown of homocysteine and prevents its high concentration in your blood. Vitamin B12 deficiency means high levels of homocysteine, which can increase your risk of atherosclerosis.

Skin darkening and hyperpigmentation: Vitamin B12 deficiency can cause unnatural skin darkening in the fingers and oral mucosa. It can also cause hyperpigmentation due to increased melanin production. Vitamin B12 deficiency leads to the oxidation of glutathione, which is essential for fighting free radicals. This affects the body's antioxidant system and leads to a decrease in the GSH/GSSG ratio. As a result, melanocytes in the skin are stimulated to produce more melanin, which causes skin darkening.

What are the symptoms of vitamin B12 deficiency?

The common symptoms and signs of vitamin B12 deficiency are given below:
- Fatigue
- Pale skin
- Shortness of breath
- Depressive feeling
- Low RBCs and WBCs
- Numbness
- Tingling sensation in the hands and feet
- Swollen tongue (glossitis of the tongue)
- Heart pounding
- Delayed development in babies
- Nerve damage (due to severe vitamin B12 deficiency)

How is vitamin B12 deficiency diagnosed?

A simple blood test can determine your vitamin B12 levels. Some standard methods to determine vitamin B12 levels are:

Serum Vitamin B12 Concentration

Vitamin B12 status is usually determined by measuring serum or plasma vitamin B12 levels. This is the most common test to assess vitamin B12 status. Normal levels and deficiency limits vary by method and laboratory. The most common level indicating vitamin B12 deficiency is

Less than 200 or 250 pg/mL (or less than 148 or 185 pmol/L): Vitamin B12 deficiency

Methylmalonic Acid (MMA) Levels

Methylmalonic acid (MMA) is a vitamin B12-associated metabolite that is the most sensitive marker of vitamin B12 status:

Serum methylmalonic acid levels greater than 0.271 µmol/L indicate vitamin B12 deficiency.

However, MMA levels are not a reliable measure because serum methylmalonic acid levels can also increase with kidney disease and aging. It is recommended that if a person's serum vitamin B12 level is between 150 and 399 pg/mL (111 to 294 pmol/L), then serum MMA levels should be checked to confirm the diagnosis of vitamin B12 deficiency.

Homocysteine Levels

Another method of determining vitamin B12 levels is to measure total plasma homocysteine levels. Vitamin B12 is involved in the breakdown of homocysteine. High levels of homocysteine mean decreased vitamin B12 levels. Serum homocysteine levels greater than 15 µmol/L indicate vitamin B12 deficiency. This method is also unreliable, as folate deficiency and kidney disease can elevate homocysteine levels.

2. IMPORTANCE OF VITAMIN B12

FUNCTIONS OF VITAMIN B12 IN THE BODY

Synthesis of DNA, RNA, And Proteins

Vitamin B12 plays a critical role in the synthesis and stability of DNA. It works as a cofactor for methionine synthase and methylmalonyl-CoA mutase enzymes. These two important enzymes are involved in DNA methylation and the synthesis of DNA and RNA. The vitamin B12-dependent enzyme methionine synthase (MS) catalyzes the conversion of homocysteine to methionine. Your body uses methionine to make proteins. During the methylation of DNA, methionine is further converted to S-adenosyl-methionine (SAM). Vitamin B12 deficiency lowers methionine and SAM levels in your body, which reduces methylation of DNA. The methylation process is essential for DNA replication and transcription, which regulate gene expression. Any deficiency in this process leads to genetic instability.

Vitamin B12 also kills free radicals through its antioxidant activities, thus protecting DNA from damage caused by oxidative stress.

Maintain Brain Health

Vitamin B12 plays a vital role in various biological events that help maintain normal neural functions. Mecobalamin, one of the active forms of vitamin B12, is crucially involved in regenerating nerves. It also enhances the formation of myelinated nerve fiber (the formation of myelin sheath), a protective layer around the brain that helps transmit information quickly and efficiently through nerve cells. It also promotes the synthesis of lecithin, which repair damaged nerve cells. Vitamin B12 increases brain-derived neurotrophic factor (BDNF) expression in injured nerves at both mRNA and protein levels, which promotes regeneration and functional recovery of injured nerves.

Vitamin B12 is an antioxidant that scavenges reactive oxygen species. It has a protective effect on neurons as it prevents nerve death caused by oxidative stress. Vitamin B12 acts as a cofactor in the synthesis of serotonin and dopamine neurotransmitters that regulate mood and sleep. Serotonin works with melatonin to regulate when you fall asleep and wake up, while dopamine energizes you and makes you feel happy.

Synthesis of Hemoglobin

Vitamin B12, as well as vitamin B6 and folate, are needed for healthy heme formation of hemoglobin, the main part of the red blood cell that gives it its red color and enables it to carry oxygen. Vitamin B12 acts as a cofactor in heme formation, which is the main part of hemoglobin. The active form of vitamin B12 is required by the enzyme that enables the conversion of L-methylmalonyl-coenzyme A to succinyl-coenzyme A (succinyl-CoA), which plays an essential role in the synthesis of heme. Hemoglobin of RBC is responsible for carrying oxygen to all your tissues and organs.

Energy Production

Vitamin B12 functions as a coenzyme in converting protein and fat into energy. The active form of vitamin B12, L-methylmalonyl-CoA mutase, converts L-methylmalonyl-CoA to succinyl-CoA. Succinyl-CoA plays an important role in the metabolism of short-chain fatty acids and amino acids. Succinyl-CoA is the entry point for propionate (a short-chain fatty acid) and valine and isoleucine (branched-chain amino acids) in the energy-producing pathway.

Maintain Homocysteine Levels

Vitamins B6, B12, and folate primarily regulate homocysteine levels. Homocysteine is the result of the essential amino acid methionine metabolism. Methionine breaks down into homocysteine. High homocysteine levels in the body are associated with an increased risk of cardiovascular disorders and stroke. Vitamin B6, vitamin B12, and folate are responsible for breaking down homocysteine into other chemicals that have vital functions in your body. Vitamin B6 is required to break down homocysteine into cysteine, while vitamin B12 and folate convert it back to methionine.

This remethylation process primarily sets the basal homocysteine levels in your body. The remethylation reaction of homocysteine to methionine is catalyzed by an enzyme called methionine synthase (MS). This enzyme requires vitamin B12 as a cofactor and a form of folate to perform its function. Without enough vitamin B12 in your body, homocysteine cannot be converted to methionine, and its levels in your blood increase, which can damage your blood vessels, including arteries and brain cells.

Antioxidant and Anti-Inflammatory Properties

Vitamin B12 exhibits antioxidant properties in several ways and protects against oxidative damage. Vitamin B12 acts as a direct antioxidant and kills free radicals in the cytosol and mitochondria. Vitamin B12 also shows strong free radical killing properties in the nervous system. Additionally, oxidative stress causes activation of apoptosis factor, which leads to cell death. Vitamin B12 inhibits the activation of the apoptosis factor and prevents cell death.

The right amount of vitamin B12 also affects the preservation of glutathione, a potent antioxidant. Vitamin B12 indirectly stimulates the deactivation of free radicals by preserving the right amount of glutathione, which is a direct antioxidant in your body's antioxidant system. The involvement of vitamin B12 in homocysteine metabolism also helps prevent oxidative stress, as excessive homocysteine leads to the formation of free radicals. It helps convert homocysteine to methionine and indirectly reduces oxidative stress in your body.

Vitamin B12 has anti-inflammatory effects as it modulates the production of inflammation-causing molecules. The pro-inflammatory cytokines IL-6 and C-reactive protein (CRP) promote inflammation in your body, increasing the levels of free radicals, which cause oxidative stress. Vitamin B12 levels and pro-inflammatory production are inversely related. Low levels of vitamin B12 make your body produce more cytokines IL-6 and high levels of this vitamin are associated with lower production of inflammation, causing cytokines IL-6 and C-reactive protein (CRP).

TOP HEALTH BENEFITS OF VITAMIN B12

1. Boost Energy and Stamina: Vitamin B12 is involved in energy and red blood cell production. Consuming a diet rich in vitamin B12 increases your energy levels, boosts your stamina, and improves your athletic performance. However, this is only true if you consume vitamin B12 through natural sources, not through supplements. Studies have not found any beneficial effects of vitamin B12 supplements on sports performance.

2. Prevent Pernicious Anemia: Pernicious anemia causes vitamin B12 deficiency, and vitamin B12 deficiency causes megaloblastic anemia. Vitamin B12 can prevent both of these anemias. Pernicious anemia is an autoimmune disorder in which your immune system secretes antibodies that block the intrinsic factor needed for vitamin B12 absorption. Pernicious anemia can be treated with intramuscular vitamin B12 injections. When vitamin B12 stores return to normal, your doctor prescribes high doses of oral vitamin B12 to maintain normal levels of this vitamin.

Similarly, megaloblastic anemia is the result of vitamin B12 deficiency. Vitamin B12 is needed for the production of healthy red blood cells and is required for hemoglobin synthesis. When your body lacks this vitamin, it cannot make enough hemoglobin, resulting in the formation of larger-than-normal red blood cells, which reduces the oxygen-carrying capacity. This leads to fatigue and weakness. Eating a diet high in vitamin B12 helps prevent anemia and increase your red blood cell production.

3. Prevent Heart Disease: Vitamin B12, along with vitamin B6, helps convert homocysteine into the essential amino acid methionine. This helps lower homocysteine levels in your blood. High levels of homocysteine are directly related to a higher risk of cardiovascular diseases as it damages blood vessels and promotes atherosclerosis. Maintaining low homocysteine levels is the key to keeping your heart healthy and functioning.

4. Increase Male Fertility: Men suffering from fertility issues should increase their intake of dietary vitamin B12 as it can increase their fertility rates. Vitamin B12 plays a part in the formation and maturation of sperm. It improves semen quality, increases sperm count, and enhances sperm motility. Apart from this, vitamin B12 helps to reduce oxidative damage and lowers inflammation, causing cytokine levels that help reduce sperm DNA damage.

5. Prevent Birth Defects: Vitamin B12 is crucial for a healthy pregnancy. High intake of vitamin B12 during pregnancy helps promote the baby's growth. It reduces the risks of miscarriage and prevents premature birth. High vitamin B12 intake, along with high folate intake, helps prevent birth defects, such as neural tube defects in the baby.

6. Mood Enhancer: Low levels of vitamin B12 are associated with depression. Vitamin B12 helps enhance your mood and reduce your stress levels. It plays a vital role as a cofactor in synthesizing mood-enhancing neurotransmitters such as serotonin and dopamine. These hormones help you calm down and feel happy.

Consuming foods high in vitamin B12 boosts your mood and emotions and helps you sleep better at night.

7. Boost Cognitive Health: Low levels of vitamin B12 are associated with higher incidences of Alzheimer's disease and dementia. Increased levels of homocysteine have a negative impact on the brain in several ways. It damages nerve cells, leading to neuronal cell death, and inhibits methylation reactions necessary for DNA and RNA synthesis. Vitamin B12 helps in the breakdown of homocysteine, thereby lowering its levels in the blood. Vitamin B12 is involved in the conversion of homocysteine back to methionine, which is an antioxidant that helps prevent oxidative damage to nerve cells. Also, vitamin B12 is necessary for RBC production, which supplies oxygen and nutrients to your brain. Eating a diet rich in vitamin B12 significantly reduces your risks of brain diseases.

8. Prevent Graying Hair: Low vitamin B12 levels can reduce hair, nails, and skin pigmentation. Vitamin B12 deficiency and sometimes high vitamin B12 levels can cause discoloration or hyperpigmentation of skin, hair, and nails. Vitamin B12 is involved in the proper production of melanin, which gives pigmentation to your hair and skin. If you are noticing premature graying of your hair, get your vitamin B12 levels checked. If you have vitamin B12 deficiency, take vitamin B12 orally as prescribed by your healthcare provider, and once it becomes normal, increase your intake of vitamin B12-rich foods.

3.
10 RICHEST VEGETARIAN SOURCES OF VITAMIN B12

Below are the top 10 vitamin B12 rich foods for vegetarians:

1. Yogurt

Eating yogurt daily is an excellent way to get more vitamin B12. Yogurt has the highest absorption of vitamin B12. A bowl of plain yogurt can fulfill 50% to 75% of the daily value of vitamin 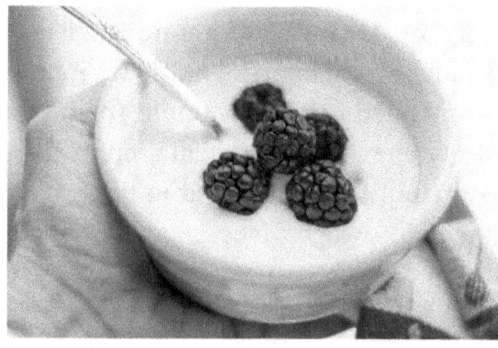 B12. It is also a good source of folate and vitamin B6. Choose low-fat and unsweetened plain yogurt to avoid weight gain.

2. Cow's Milk

Milk is another excellent source of vitamin B12, and adequate consumption may help prevent vitamin B12 deficiency. About 2 cups of 250 ml of milk per day can get

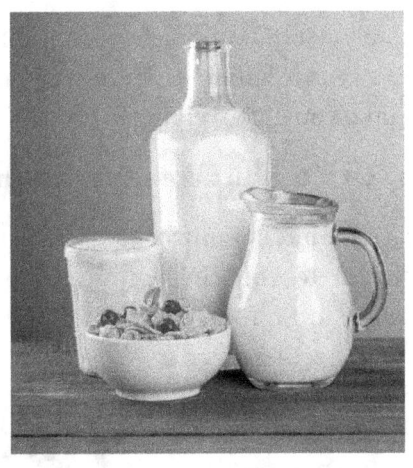

you the recommended daily intake of vitamin B12. It is loaded with other nutrients such as calcium, protein, potassium, and phosphorus. Consuming it with breakfast cereal, which is usually fortified with essential vitamins, can increase vitamin B12 levels in your body.

3. Cheese

Cheese is a fair source of vitamin B12. Some varieties of cheese, such as Swiss cheese, cottage cheese (paneer), and mozzarella cheese, are high in vitamin B12. Avoid processed cheese, as the amount of vitamin B12 is very low in it. One slice of cheese

is enough to provide you with 22% to 36% of the recommended daily intake of vitamin B12, but do not solely depend upon cheese to fulfill your daily vitamin B12 requirement, as large consumption of cheese may make you gain weight.

4. Dried Shiitake Mushroom

Dried Shiitake mushrooms, a type of fungi, have been shown to contain significant levels of vitamin B12. These are not an excellent source of vitamin B12, but they are decent. Shiitake mushrooms do not naturally produce vitamin B12; the vitamin B12 found in dried shiitake 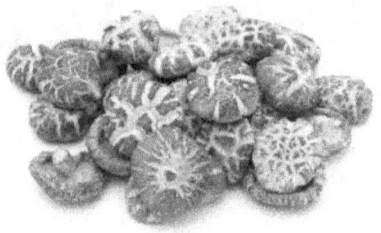 mushrooms is derived from the bed logs in which they are grown. You can increase your overall vitamin B12 intake by adding dried shiitake mushrooms, tempeh, and cheese to your wraps and stuffing. 50 g of dried Shiitake mushrooms fulfils 100% of your daily vitamin B12 requirement.

5. Whey Protein

Whey protein is a great source of vitamin B12. You can make your own whey protein at home by curdling boiled milk with lemon juice. The liquid part of this process is your whey, which is rich in vitamin B12 and a great source of protein for vegetarians. Use this whey in your pancake batter or add it to your pasta recipes to get the full health benefits of whey.

6. Vanilla Ice Cream

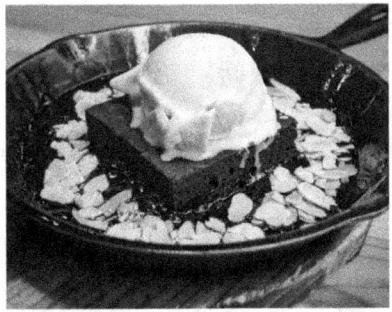

Ice cream is made of milk, and vitamin B12 is naturally found in milk, making ice cream a good source of vitamin B12. It also contains vitamins A, C, D, K, and E, as well as calcium and protein. However, ice cream is high in cholesterol and saturated fat. Therefore, it should be consumed in a lesser amount for overall health. A single cup serving of vanilla ice cream has 20 % of the daily recommended intake of vitamin B12.

7. Chlorella

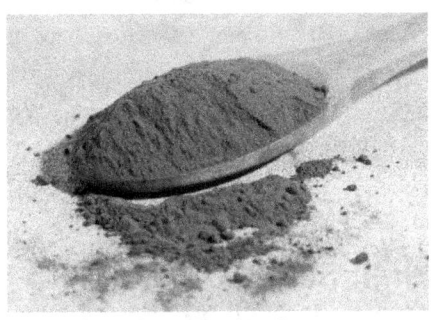

Chlorella is green algae that grows in fresh water. It is considered vegetarian and is sometimes referred to as seaweed. Unlike plant-based food sources, chlorella contains vitamin B12 as well as vitamin D. It also contains higher amounts of iron and folate than plant-based foods. However, the problem is that the amount of vitamin B12 in chlorella depends on the growing conditions and the presence of microorganisms around the algae. Vitamin B12 is not produced by chlorella but by microorganisms living in the soil or the plant in fresh water. Nori, another seaweed, is also a rich source of vitamin B12 but has the same limitations as chlorella. Additionally, studies show that the process of drying nori robs it of its vitamin B12 content.

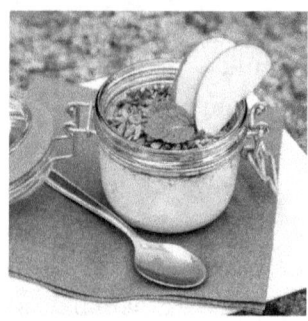

8. Probiotic Foods

Your body can make some vitamin B12, which contributes to its status. Lactobacillus and Bifidobacterium bacteria species can form vitamin B12 in your gut. Foods containing Lactobacillus and Bifidobacterium can help increase your vitamin B12 level. Probiotics are known to increase the growth of good bacteria in your gut, contributing to vitamin B12 production in your body. Yogurt is the best example of a probiotic. Some fruits that are natural probiotics are bananas, watermelon, custard apples, apples, and grapefruit. Some of these fruits also have prebiotic properties, meaning they act as a food source for the bacteria in your gut and increase the growth and production of gut bacteria, which contributes to the increased production of vitamin B12 in your body.

9. Fermented Foods

Consuming fermented foods is associated with higher concentrations of vitamin B12 in your body. Fermented foods can be sources of Lactobacillus and Bifidobacterium, which have vitamin B12-producing ability with their probiotic potential. The fermentation process involves microbial growth that produces fermented products. When consumed by humans, these good microorganisms in fermented products act as probiotics and support vitamin B12-producing bacteria in your gut. Some good examples of fermented foods around the world are idli, dosa, dhokla, khaman, kefir, kimchi, tempeh, miso, sauerkraut, and kombucha.

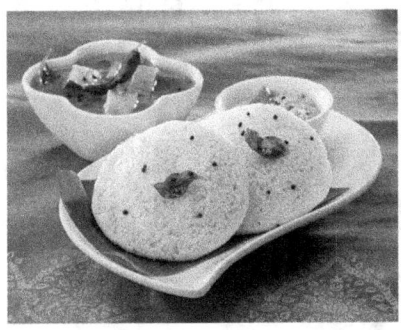

10. Cobalt Rich Foods

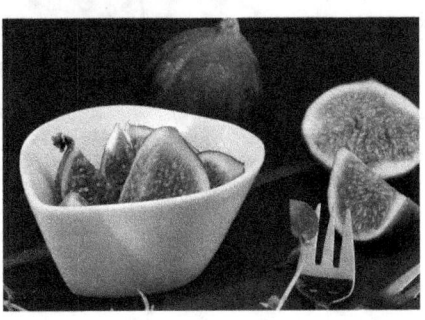

Cobalt is a key part of vitamin B12's structure. It is a trace mineral that microorganisms in your gut require to manufacture vitamin B12. Low cobalt levels in your body may hinder the formation of essential vitamin B12. Therefore, if you get enough cobalt, you increase the production of vitamin B12 in your gut. Some good food sources of cobalt are green leafy vegetables, like spinach and broccoli, milk, figs, dates, raisins, plums, apricots, oats, and drinking water.

UNIT 3
VITAMIN C

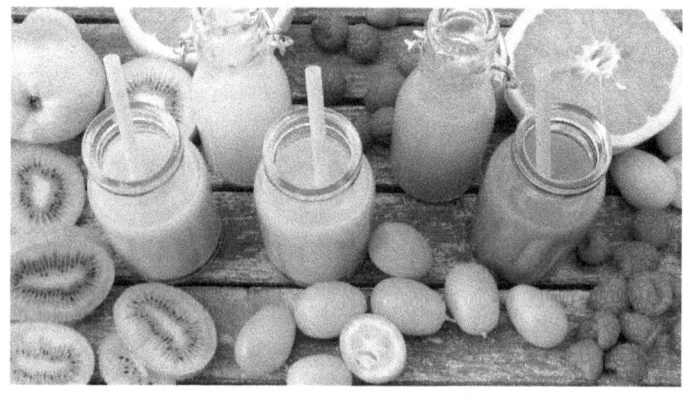

1.
EVERYTHING YOU NEED TO KNOW ABOUT VITAMIN C

What is vitamin C, and what does it do?

Vitamin C is an essential water-soluble vitamin, which is also known as ascorbic acid. Your body cannot synthesize ascorbic acid alone; therefore, it must be obtained from food. Vitamin C plays an irreplaceable role in boosting immune response and fighting infections. It is also crucial in forming a protein called collagen, which plays an essential role in wound healing.

How is vitamin C metabolized in the body?

Vitamin C is well absorbed in your body. It is absorbed in the small intestine and is regulated by active transporters. Dehydroascorbic acid is a form of vitamin C found in vitamin C supplements. It is the oxidized form of vitamin C. Glucose transporters facilitate the entry of dehydroascorbic acid into cells, which is then converted into ascorbic acid in your body.

The absorption of vitamin C in your body depends on the amount of vitamin C consumed. Eating more vitamin C does not necessarily mean you are getting more vitamin C. When you consume moderate amounts of 30-180 mg of vitamin C a day, about 70%-90% of the vitamin C is absorbed. However, higher intakes of 1 gram or 1000 mg per day decrease absorption, and absorption is reduced to less than 50% and excreted in the urine. In fact, doses as high as 3 g thrice daily may not increase the absorption rate, and the actual amount of vitamin C that reaches your blood circulation is much less than what typically reaches at such high levels (220 μmol/L).

Your body maintains high levels of vitamin C in cells and tissues. The higher levels of vitamin C are found in the white blood cells (WBCs), eyes, pituitary gland, adrenal glands, and brain, and the lower levels are found in red blood cells (RBCs), plasma, and saliva (in the extracellular fluid).

Is vitamin C stored in the body?

Unlike fat-soluble vitamins, vitamin C is not stored in your body for long and is excreted through urine, so it is important to take it daily.

Is vitamin C really an essential nutrient?

Yes, vitamin C is an essential vitamin because your body cannot make it. Your body requires a constant supply of vitamin C through dietary sources every day.

Do heat and light destroy vitamin C?

Vitamin C is sensitive to ligh tand heat. This means that high temperatures and exposure to light destroy vitamin C. Prolonged cooking of vitamin C foods at a high temperature can destroy this vitamin. It is best to take vitamin C in raw form as fully ripped foods contain maximum vitamin C. If you cook vitamin C food in water, it leaches out into the liquid, so it is best to consume the liquid portion, as most of the vitamin C is available in this portion. It is best to stir-fry or blanch vitamin C-rich foods for a short time to retain their vitamin C content while cooking.

Vitamin C is unstable and easily oxidized in light. So, exposing your vitamin C-rich foods to light significantly reduces their vitamin C content.

How much vitamin C do I need?

The Recommended Dietary Allowance (RDA) for vitamin C is not based on the amount needed to protect against vitamin C deficiency; in fact, it is much higher than that. The recommended intake is based on its known physiological requirements and antioxidant functions in white blood cells. The average daily level of vitamin C sufficient to meet the physiological needs of healthy individuals is given below:

Age	Male	Female
0–6 m	40 mg*	40 mg*
7–12 m	50 mg*	50 mg*
1–3 yrs.	15 mg	15 mg
4–8 yrs.	25 mg	25 mg
9–13 yrs.	45 mg	45 mg
14–18 yrs.	75 mg	65 mg
19+ yrs.	90 mg	75 mg

* Adequate Intake (AI)

**People who smoke need 35 mg/day more vitamin C than non-smokers.

What happens if I have a vitamin C deficiency?

Vitamin C deficiency can lead to the following health problems:

Scurvy: Severe vitamin C deficiency causes scurvy. Vitamin C is essential for collagen formation. Vitamin C deficiency causes collagen loss, which weakens connective tissue, blood vessels, and bones. Scurvy has symptoms of collagen deficiency, such as poor wound healing, bleeding and easy bruising, joint pain, hair loss, tooth decay, and fatigue.

Cancer: Patients with advanced cancer are often found to have low levels of vitamin C. Although there is no direct link between vitamin C deficiency and cancer, vitamin C acts as an antioxidant and protects DNA from oxidative damage, helping to keep the risk of cancer to a minimum. Therefore, a deficiency of vitamin C lowers your body's defenses and may put you at risk of developing cancer.

Heart diseases: Vitamin C helps prevent heart attacks by protecting your blood vessels from free radicals-induced damage, thus reducing atherosclerosis risk. Vitamin C deficiency reduces your body's antioxidant defense system, and your body cannot protect the blood vessels from oxidative damage by free radicals, which increases the risk of heart disease.

What are the symptoms of vitamin C deficiency?

Vitamin C deficiency is associated with the following signs and symptoms:

- Lack of energy
- Fatigue
- Muscular pain
- Pain in joints
- Weight loss
- Coiled hair
- Swollen gums
- Poor wound healing

What factors can be responsible for vitamin C deficiency?

Smoking: It is scientifically proven that people who smoke have lower vitamin C levels than non-smokers. This is because smoking increases oxidative stress and reduces vitamin C levels. Therefore, smokers need more vitamin C to meet the increased demand of their bodies. Smokers require 35 mg more vitamin C per day than non-smokers. Even if you do not smoke but are regularly exposed to cigarette smoke, your vitamin C levels may be low. Passive smokers require more vitamin C than people who are not exposed to cigarette smoke.

Alcohol dependence: Alcohol significantly increases the excretion of vitamin C in the urine, which can cause vitamin C deficiency, especially in people who are addicted to alcohol. Alcohol addiction can also cause chronic diarrhea, which results in poor absorption and makes your body unable to absorb the vitamin C you eat. This eventually leads to vitamin C deficiency.

Drug addiction: Constant drug abuse has a negative effect on levels of vitamin C in the body, leading to vitamin C deficiency over time. People who are drug addicts have low levels of vitamin C. Due to the lack of vitamin C in the body, it cannot fulfill its antioxidant protective function. This makes the body vulnerable to other chronic diseases.

Feeding boiled cow milk to infants: It is not advised to feed boiled cow milk to infants. Mother's milk contains an adequate amount of vitamin C, while cow's milk naturally contains very little vitamin C. Since vitamin C degrades in heat, boiling cow's milk destroys vitamin C.

Consumption of a limited variety of foods: People who follow a restricted diet that is not scientifically proven tend to limit their intake of a variety of foods. Vitamin C is primarily derived from fruits and vegetables, but a varied diet is necessary to meet the recommended amount of vitamin C in a day. Following a certain diet that allows only certain types of nutrients while restricting other nutrients can lead to nutrient deficiencies that are not limited to vitamin C.

Malabsorption: Malabsorption is a condition that impairs the absorption of nutrients through the small intestine. Malabsorption can be caused by infections, small intestine surgery, certain medications such as tetracycline, antacids, drugs to treat obesity, and certain disorders such as celiac disease.

Certain medical conditions: Certain medical conditions can decrease vitamin C levels or increase the demand needed by the body. Vitamin C concentrations may be low in patients with dialysis, cachexia, and cancer.

What happens if I take too much vitamin C?

Vitamin C from dietary sources does not cause any side effects. Taking high doses of vitamin C supplements may cause toxicity and some adverse effects, such as nausea, diarrhea, and stomach cramps. High intakes of vitamin C reduce the levels of vitamin B12 and copper in your body. Vitamin C at high levels may act as a pro-oxidant and cause oxidative damage to DNA and chromosomes that potentially contribute to cancer development. The upper limit (UL) of vitamin C for adults is 2,000 mg per day. However, this upper limit does not apply to people taking vitamin C for medical treatment under the supervision of a physician.

How is vitamin C deficiency diagnosed?

Vitamin C deficiency is diagnosed by a physical examination. Physicians usually check for signs of skin or gum disease. A complete blood count (CBC) is performed to detect anemia if necessary. Bleeding, coagulation, as well as prothrombin time are also checked if necessary.

Scurvy is initially diagnosed based on the symptoms, and measuring vitamin C levels in plasma or serum through a simple blood test can confirm the diagnosis. A vitamin C level of less than 0.2 mg/dL (10 µmol/L) indicates severe deficiency. It is confirmed through a skin biopsy to check for coiled hair follicles, hyperkeratosis, perifollicular bleeding, and proliferation of blood vessels.

2.
IMPORTANCE OF VITAMIN C

FUNCTIONS OF ASCORBIC ACID IN THE BODY

Antioxidant Functions

Free radicals are formed when your body breaks down food to convert it into energy. Fewer free radicals are not harmful and can be neutralized by your body's antioxidants. But when free radicals exceed the antioxidants in your body, they start pairing with lipids, proteins, and DNA. This oxidation of lipids, proteins, and DNA damages them and puts you at risk of cancer, heart disease, and stroke. Diseases like atherosclerosis and cancer are caused by oxidant damage to tissues.

In today's lifestyle, free radicals are produced not only by your body but also in large amounts when exposed to cigarette smoke, X-rays, and radiation from the sun.

Eating foods high in antioxidants is essential to neutralize these increased free radicals. Vitamin C is a potent water-soluble antioxidant. It helps protect cells and tissues from the harmful effects of free radicals. Vitamin C acts as both a direct and indirect antioxidant. It directly neutralizes free radicals and prevents some of the damage they cause. Despite being a water-soluble antioxidant, vitamin C protects membranes and hydrophobic compartments from free radical damage by regenerating the fat-soluble antioxidant vitamin E within the body.

Vitamin C helps recycle vitamin E. After vitamin E binds to free radicals to neutralize them, it itself becomes oxidized and cannot bind further to other free radicals. When your body has enough vitamin C, it reduces oxidized vitamin E back to its original form. When restored, vitamin E can bind to free radicals again, rendering them ineffective. Together, vitamins C and E form an antioxidant network that protects against chronic diseases by protecting lipids, proteins, and DNA from free radical damage.

Interestingly, research studies have found that long-term high doses of vitamin C, about 500 mg per day for up to 6 weeks, can exhibit antioxidant as well as prooxidant effects. This means vitamin C can cause oxidative damage to DNA in high doses. This is only possible with vitamin C supplements, not when you get it from fruits and vegetables. This effect is reversible; it stops when you stop taking high-dose vitamin C supplements. However, alcoholics should be extra careful as vitamin C participates in ethanol metabolism and produces highly reactive radicals, so caution should be exercised even if you are a moderate drinker.

> *Read Eat So What! The Science of Fat-Soluble Vitamins to understand oxidative stress, free radicals, and oxidant damage in detail.*

Collagen Formation and Role of Collagen in the Body

Collagen is the structural protein found in the highest amount in the body. It is essential for maintaining the integrity and strength of connective tissues. Collagen is rigid and resistant to stretch, making it the primary building block of bones, skin, muscles, ligaments, tendons, and other connective tissues.

Connective tissue is a group of tissues found in the highest amount throughout the body and maintains the shape of the body and organs. As the name suggests, it links various tissues in the body and is a significant component of skin, bone, tendons, and muscles.

Collagen is responsible for your skin's structure, elasticity, and strength. It helps replace dead skin cells and grow new cells. It forms a protective covering over organs and aids blood clotting during wound healing.

Vitamin C is essential for collagen formation. It has a significant role in maintaining a standard collagen network in the body and regulates collagen synthesis. Vitamin C aids in collagen biosynthesis by preventing the auto-inactivation of two key enzymes, lysyl and prolyl hydroxylase, thus maintaining a typical collagen network in the body.

Maintaining Immune Function

Vitamin C has an essential role in immune defense. It supports the cellular functions of both the adaptive and innate immune systems. It contributes to immune defense through its potent antioxidant activities and acts as a gene regulatory enzyme cofactor. It stimulates white blood cell activity.

During microbial infection, vitamin C accumulates in phagocytic cells and enhances phagocytosis, a cellular process of engulfing and ultimately killing bacteria.

Vitamin C promotes the skin's oxidant scavenging activity and protects against environmental oxidative stress. It also supports the skin's epithelial barrier function and prevents pathogen attack.

TOP HEALTH BENEFITS OF VITAMIN C

1. Wound Healing: Vitamin C is important in all phases of wound healing. It promotes the regenerative process, thereby accelerating recovery. It decreases inflammatory mediators and increases healing mediators.

In the inflammatory phase, vitamin C aids in neutrophil apoptosis and clearance. Vitamin C is required for collagen synthesis, maturation, secretion, and its degradation during the proliferative phase.

The healing of bone, tendons, and ligaments depends on the capacity and efficiency of collagen synthesis and cross-linking. Inadequate collagen formation results in poorly developed extracellular matrix, which may lead to inadequate tissue structures and affect their strength, resulting in an increased risk of re-injury. Vitamin C enhances collagen synthesis and soft tissue healing.

Vitamin C also aids in wound healing through its antioxidant action. Wound healing increases the production of free radicals, which can cause tissue damage and delayed healing. Vitamin C acts as an antioxidant; it reduces oxidative stress and inflammation by scavenging these reactive oxygen species. Vitamin C reduces tissue damage and speeds up the wound-healing process by reducing the harmful effects of free radicals.

2. Prevent Scurvy: Eating enough vitamin C-rich foods helps prevent scurvy. Scurvy is caused by inadequate intake of vitamin C and includes fatigue or lethargy and bleeding gums. As vitamin C deficiency progresses, it negatively affects collagen formation, resulting in weak connective tissue, leading to joint pain, poor wound healing, corkscrew hair, and thick and rough patches on the skin. Even acute vitamin C deficiency can lead to scurvy and can cause death if left untreated. Although cases of scurvy are now rare, it can still occur in people who do not eat enough fruits and vegetables.

3. Absorption of Nonheme Iron: Your body absorbs two types of iron from food. Heme iron is present in animal-based products such as seafood, meat, poultry, and fish, while nonheme iron comes from plant foods such as grains, fruits, beans, vegetables, nuts, and seeds. Heme iron is better absorbed by the body than nonheme but may increase the risk of cancer, heart disease, and stroke.

Nonheme iron is the primary type of iron for humans, but it is not well absorbed by the body, and its absorption is highly affected by other foods consumed in the same meal. Foods containing tannins, calcium, phosphate, phytates, and polyphenols reduce iron absorption in your body. Tannins containing foods such as tea and coffee, calcium and phosphate-rich foods such as dairy products, and phytates in cereals, nuts, and seeds reduce iron absorption in the body.

Vitamin C is a potent nonheme iron absorption enhancer that reverses the inhibitory effects of tea and calcium/phosphate-rich foods.

Vitamin C forms a chelate with ferric iron at the acid pH of the stomach, keeping the iron soluble at the alkaline pH of the small intestine. Eat iron-rich foods with vitamin C-rich foods in the same meal for better iron absorption in your body.

4. Cancer Prevention: Vitamin C intake is inversely related to various types of cancer, including breast, lung, stomach, and colon cancer. It has been found that people suffering from cancer have low levels of vitamin C. High vitamin C intake prevents the risk of cancer. It limits the formation of carcinogens such as nitrosamines, regulates the immune response, and reduces oxidative damage to cells and tissues through its antioxidant activity.

However, this cancer-preventing effect is only possible if you get vitamin C from fruits and vegetables, not supplements. Results from several clinical trials suggest that vitamin C supplementation provides no benefit in cancer prevention.

5. Prevention of Heart Disease: A high dietary intake of vitamin C is associated with a lower risk of heart disease. This is mainly due to its antioxidant activity. Vitamin C prevents the deposition of cholesterol and, therefore, prevents heart attacks.

Oxidative damage to low-density lipoproteins is a major cause of heart disease. It builds up as plaque in the arteries and may result in stroke or heart attack. Vitamin C, through its antioxidant properties, prevents oxidative damage to LDL cholesterol and cardiovascular diseases.

In addition, vitamin C contributes to heart health by reducing high blood pressure. It improves vasodilation, increases nitric oxide production, and reduces vascular smooth muscle cell apoptosis.

People who have low vitamin C levels are at risk of heart attack and stroke, although vitamin C intake does not reduce mortality due to heart disease. In fact, intake of vitamin C supplements of about 300 mg per day may even increase mortality, especially in older women who have diabetes.

6. Prevent Age-Related Vision Diseases: Cataracts and age-related macular degeneration (AMD) are two significant causes of vision loss in elderly people. One of the major causes of these diseases is oxidative stress. Vitamin C is a powerful antioxidant that reduces oxidative damage and significantly affects the development and treatment of these diseases.

Higher dietary intake of vitamin C is associated with a reduced risk of cataract formation and slower progression of AMD. Recent research studies do not prove vitamin C's role in preventing age-related macular degeneration, but several studies strongly suggest that it may help slow the progression of age-related macular degeneration. Vitamin C from fruits and vegetables helps prevent cataracts. However, vitamin C supplements fail to produce the same effect. In fact, intake of high-dose vitamin C supplements is associated with a 25% higher risk of age-related cataract disease.

7. Promotes Mental Vitality: Vitality means a feeling of energy and vivacity. Vitamin C promotes mental vitality, it contributes to better performance on cognitive activities by increasing motivation and the ability to concentrate.

You will be surprised to know that vitamin C is present in the highest concentrations in the brain. It plays a vital role in brain functions and maintaining normal mental health. Vitamin C has antioxidant and neuro-modulating effects on neurotransmitters in your brain. Through its antioxidant activity, vitamin C protects neurons from oxidative damage and induces differentiation and maturation of neurons. It regulates the synthesis of neuro-modulating agents, including serotonin, catecholamines, and glutamate. It enhances serotonin release and has a relieving effect on anxious moods.

Vitamin C deficiency leads to decreased physical activity and altered social behavior. This is due to the interaction of vitamin C with the dopaminergic system. Vitamin C enhances dopaminergic signaling and helps convert dopamine to a norepinephrine transmitter. Low levels of norepinephrine lead to feelings of depression or anxiety. Dopaminergic signaling is positively associated with emotional arousal, such as motivation, self-control, attention, and improved cognitive performance.

8. Prevent Motion Sickness: You may have experienced motion sickness while traveling in a car, airplane, boat, amusement park ride, or at high altitude. Motion sickness occurs when your brain receives conflicting signals from your eyes, inner ear, and the body. Your brain cannot handle these mixed signals, and you feel dizzy, nauseated, and vomit. This triggers histamine release, which controls vomiting reactions. Vitamin C has strong antihistamine properties. It is effective in suppressing the symptoms of motion sickness. It reduces the inner ear's ability to sense motion and blocks signals to the part of the brain that controls nausea and vomiting.

3.
10 RICHEST VEGETARIAN SOURCES OF VITAMIN C

Below are the 10 richest vegetarian sources of Vitamin C (Ascorbic Acid):

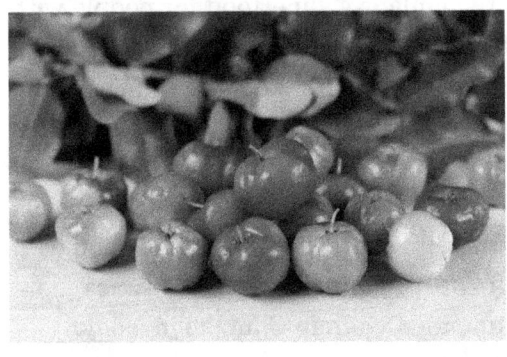

1. Acerola or West Indian Cherry

West Indian cherry, also known as Barbados cherry, is the richest source of vitamin C. 100 g of West Indian cherry contains 1680 mg of vitamin C, 18 times more than the daily recommended 90 mg of vitamin C. In fact, partially ripe acerola can contain up to 45007 mg of vitamin C per 100 grams. Acerola fruit is rich in vitamin C, carotene, vitamins B1, B2, and B3, proteins, and minerals such as iron, calcium, and phosphorus. Acerola cherry is very effective in normalizing gallbladder irregularities. Acerola has also shown active anti-fungal activities and can be used to treat colds and flu, pulmonary disorders, and liver diseases. Acerola cherry has potent antioxidant activity due to its high vitamin C content.

2. Indian gooseberry/Amla

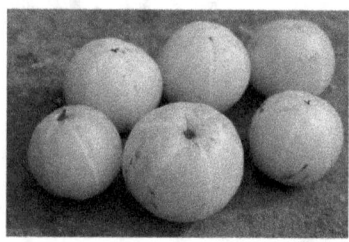

Indian gooseberry/Amla is a great source of vitamin C. It boosts immunity, aids digestion, and promotes hair growth. Most importantly, amla is a superfood for people with diabetes. Amla is highly effective in managing blood glucose levels. The vitamin C in amla helps in collagen production and enhances skin health. Indian gooseberry is rich in phenolic and flavonoid compounds that have antioxidant and antimicrobial activities. One Indian gooseberry can provide you with about 600 to 700 mg of vitamin C, seven times more than the recommended vitamin C intake in a day.

3. Bell Peppers

All types of bell peppers, red, orange, yellow, and green, contain vitamin C, but the amount varies greatly. You may be surprised to know that the most common green bell pepper has the lowest amount of vitamin C among all types of bell peppers. As bell peppers mature, they become more nutritious; green bell peppers are the unripe variety and are harvested early; they are more bitter and less sweet than other types of bell peppers. According to data published by USDA in 2022, 100 grams of raw orange bell pepper (158 mg) contains the highest amount of vitamin C, followed by red bell pepper (142 mg), yellow bell pepper (139 mg), and lastly, green bell pepper (99.5 mg).

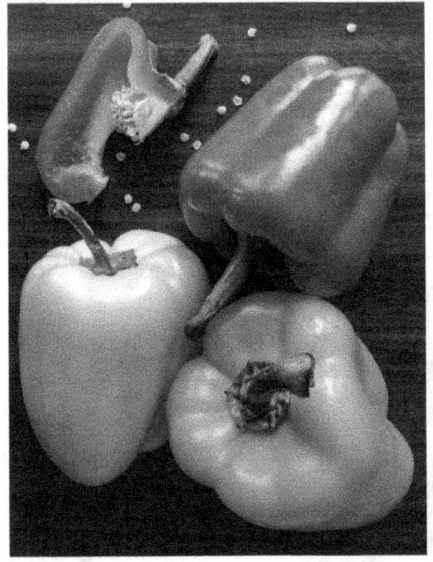

4. Guava

Guava is one of the greatest sources of vitamin C. One fruit can provide you with more than the recommended amount of vitamin C. About 55 grams of guava fruit contains 125 mg of vitamin C, and 100 g contains 228 mg of vitamin C. Not only the fruit but guava leaves are also very nutritious. Apart from boosting your immunity, guava fruits

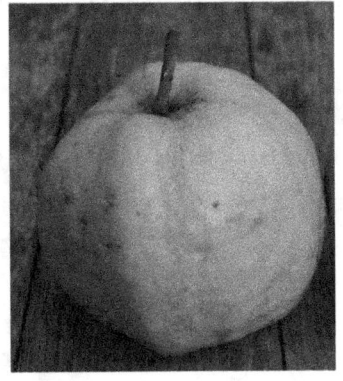

and leaves can help lower blood pressure levels and sugar levels. They have anti-cancer properties, promote gut health, and are also great for your hair and skin.

5. Blackcurrants

Blackcurrants are rich in antioxidants. They are a great source of vitamin C and anthocyanin, a flavonoid that gives blackcurrants their deep purple color. The high amounts of antioxidants present in them helps prevent tumors and heart diseases. Vitamin C acts as a free radical scavenger and prevents the formation of cancer-causing compounds in the stomach. The high vitamin C in blackcurrants has neuroprotective effects and protects the brain from damage and stroke, while anthocyanins have anti-inflammatory and antimicrobial effects and help maintain eye health. Just 20 grams of this fruit gives you the recommended daily allowance for vitamin C, as 100 grams of blackcurrant contains 160-285 mg of vitamin C.

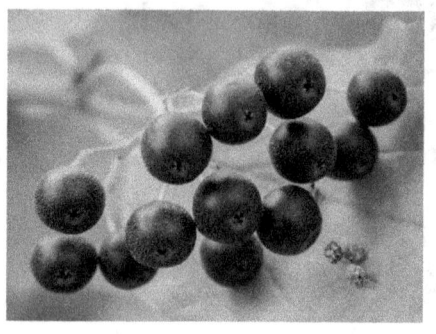

6. Kiwi

Kiwi is an outstanding source of vitamin C. Golden kiwi has a higher amount of vitamin C than green kiwi. If you want to get maximum vitamin C from kiwi, eat it with the peel. In fact, kiwi fruit peel not only contains vitamin C but also has more antioxidants than the fruit itself. It is also a good source of vitamin E, flavonoids, and fiber. Eating kiwi fruit with its peel can increase your vitamin C, vitamin E, folate, and fiber intake by up to 50%. Kiwi peel is completely edible;

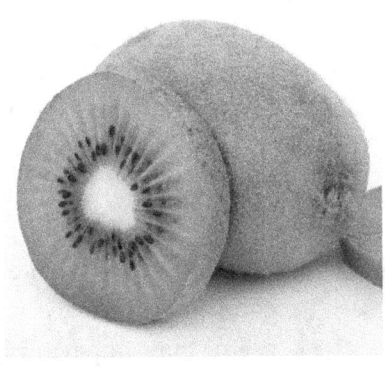

just wash them thoroughly and use them with the peel in your recipes, or eat them whole. One and a half medium-sized green kiwi fruit or one whole golden kiwi fruit can meet your daily requirement of vitamin C. 100 g of green kiwi contains 93 mg of vitamin C, while 100 grams of golden kiwi contains 161 mg of vitamin C.

7. Broccoli

Broccoli has almost twice the amount of vitamin C as compared to oranges. 100 g of broccoli contains 90 grams of vitamin C, while 100 g of oranges contains 53 g of vitamin C. However, cooking reduces the amount of vitamin C in broccoli to some extent.

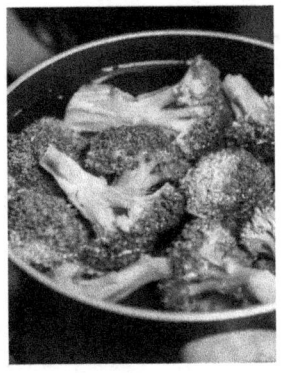

100 g of cooked broccoli contains 65 grams of vitamin C. Out of boiling, microwaving, steaming, and baking, steaming is the best way to cook broccoli to retain maximum vitamin C. Broccoli not only fulfills your vitamin C requirement but also contains many other nutrients. Broccoli is high in vitamin K, which is good for clotting and bones. The antioxidants present in broccoli can protect you from various chronic diseases.

8. Papaya

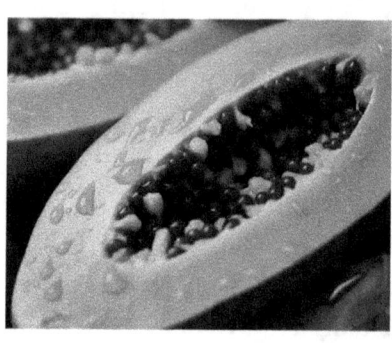

The bright orange color may make it seem that papaya is only a good source of vitamin A, but surprisingly, papaya is also an excellent source of vitamin C and folate. 100 grams of papaya contains 61 mg of vitamin C, which can meet 68% of your daily requirement. The high antioxidant vitamins A and C present in papaya help reduce the risk of heart diseases and inflammatory diseases. Not only this, papaya is also great for digestion. A special enzyme found in papaya called papain enzyme aids digestion by making proteins easily digestible. Papaya is great for relieving constipation.

9. Strawberry

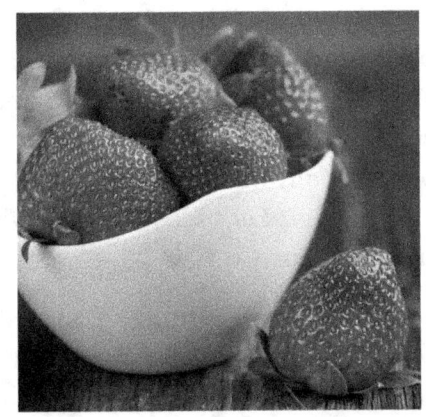

Strawberries are a nutrient-rich fruit. It is a good source of vitamin C, antioxidants, and manganese. Strawberries contain almost 90% water and have very low calories, which makes them a weight-loss-friendly fruit. Strawberries boost your immunity and reduce the chances of getting sick. Its high antioxidant content reduces inflammation and helps lower blood sugar levels and cholesterol levels. This reduces the risks of diabetes, stroke, and heart disease. 100 g of strawberries contain 58.8 mg of vitamin C, which can fulfill 65% of your daily vitamin C requirement.

10. Citrus Fruits

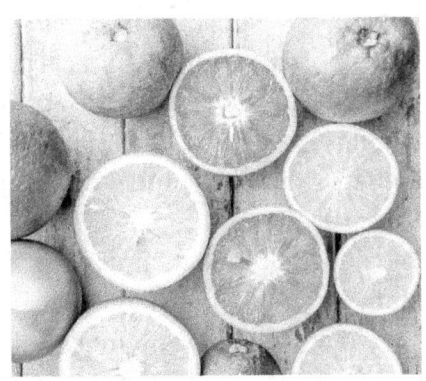

Orange | Lemon | Lime | Pineapple | Grapefruit | Pomelo

When it comes to vitamin C, the first thing that comes to mind is citrus fruits, especially oranges. Citrus fruits are definitely a rich source of vitamin C, but not the richest source. Citrus fruits are famous for vitamin C because they are very common and easily available around the world. The most common citrus fruit that comes to mind first for vitamin C is orange, but is orange really the richest source of vitamin C among all citrus fruits? Let's see how much vitamin C each citrus fruit contains.

100 g of orange contains 53.2 mg of vitamin C.
100 g of lemon contains 53 mg of vitamin C.
100 g of lime contains 29.1 mg of vitamin C.
100 g of pineapple contains 29.1 mg of vitamin C.
100 g of grapefruit contains 47.8 mg of vitamin C.
100 g of pomelo contains 61 mg of vitamin C.

So, pomelo is definitely the winner, but that doesn't mean you can't get your vitamin C from oranges. A medium-sized orange, weighing about 155 grams, can provide 93% of the vitamin C you need in a day.

OTHER HIGH VITAMIN C RICH FOODS

Other notable high vitamin C-rich that are not readily available are rose hips, which contain about 426 mg of vitamin C per 100 g, and Kakadu plums, which have the highest vitamin C content of 3 grams per 100 g of fruit. However, Kakadu plums are also very high in oxalate. People who have inflammatory diseases, a history of kidney stones, or a family history of kidney stones should avoid Kakadu plums. This is because they are high in oxalate and vitamin C, which can cause kidney

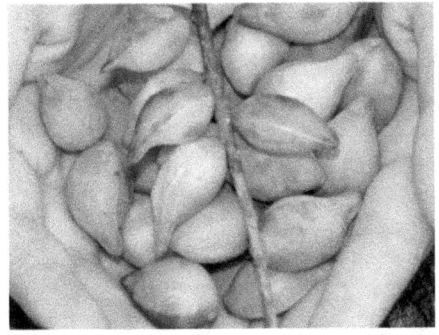
stones. Oxalate interferes with calcium absorption in the body and results in kidney stone formation.

The rosehip is located just below the petals of the rose flower and contains the seeds of the rose plant. It is high in vitamin C and is mainly used to reduce pain associated with osteoarthritis. The vitamin C content in rosehips ranges from 106 to 2712 mg per 100 g depending on the species, variety, and altitude. The Rosa nitidula variety harvested from high altitudes contains more vitamin C than other varieties at lower altitudes, but most of the vitamin C is lost during the drying of the plant.

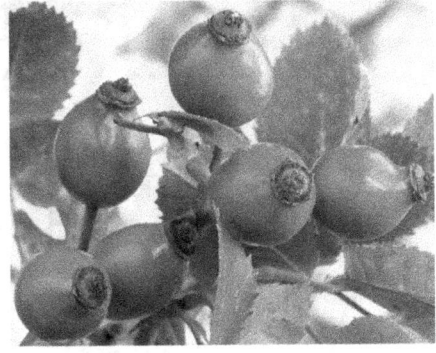

Make herbal tea using fresh rosehips to get the maximum health benefits of vitamin C.

Other decent sources of vitamin C are cauliflower, cabbage, tomatoes, potatoes, and cantaloupe.

UNIT 4
VITAMIN COMBINATIONS - DOS AND DON'TS

When taking vitamins, it's important to consider how different combinations can affect your body. For vitamins to produce their intended effects, they must be adequately absorbed into your body. Combining certain vitamins with other vitamins and minerals can increase or inhibit their absorption rate. Some vitamin combinations can have a synergistic effect, increasing the absorption of other vitamins and providing better health benefits than taking either alone. However, other combinations can interfere with their absorption into the body, nullifying their effects and potentially causing toxicity.

Let's take a look at beneficial and dangerous combinations of vitamins that can affect your health in many ways:

VITAMIN COMBINATIONS FOR SYNERGISTIC HEALTH BENEFITS

VITAMIN C AND VITAMIN E

Both vitamin C and vitamin E have strong antioxidant properties. Vitamin E is a fat-soluble antioxidant, while vitamin C is a water-soluble antioxidant. When combined, these two vitamins can boost immunity, protect against exercise-induced damage, and reduce the risk of chronic diseases. Vitamin C helps regenerate vitamin E from its inactive oxidized form. Vitamin C enhances the antioxidant action of vitamin E, making it more efficient. These vitamins are more potent when combined than when used alone. For maximum health benefits, include vitamin C-rich foods such as citrus fruits, bell peppers, and tomatoes in your diet, as well as vitamin E-rich foods such as almonds, sunflower oil, and red bell peppers. However, taking fat-soluble vitamins like vitamin E and water-soluble vitamins is not advised. Therefore, maintain a gap of 2-3 hours between the intake of both types of vitamins.

VITAMIN B5 AND VITAMIN C

Vitamin C enhances the synthesis of collagen protein and repairs damaged tissues. Vitamin C has potent free radical scavenging properties, which help reduce oxidative stress as well as inflammation, enabling an optimal environment for wound healing and accelerating the healing process. Vitamin B5 has a moisturizing effect on your skin and enhances your skin's barrier function. Vitamin C, when combined with vitamin B5, can accelerate wound healing, especially after surgery.

FOLATE AND IRON

While iron is essential for hemoglobin formation, which enables red blood cells to carry oxygen, folate is required to produce red blood cells. Iron and folate together increase hemoglobin production and support healthy red blood cell formation, which helps prevent and treat anemia. This is why iron is used along with folic acid supplements to treat anemia. Sometimes iron and folate are also prescribed in combination with vitamin B12, which helps increase red blood cell production.

VITAMIN B6 AND VITAMIN B9 WITH CALCIUM

Imbalance in hormones, neurotransmitters, and calcium regulation are some of the causes of premenstrual syndrome. Vitamin B6 can effectively reduce the emotional disturbance symptoms of premenstrual syndrome. Folate helps correct the hormonal imbalance and regulate the menstrual cycle, and calcium induces calcium balance in your body. It has been found that a combination of calcium and vitamin B6 reduces the symptoms of premenstrual syndrome better than vitamin B6 alone. Eating vitamin B6-rich foods along with folate and calcium-rich foods can better control the symptoms of premenstrual syndrome.

FOLATE AND VITAMIN C

Consuming foods high in folates, such as green leafy vegetables, black-eyed peas, and asparagus with vitamin C-rich citrus fruits, increases the efficiency of folate in your body. Vitamin C is a potent antioxidant that protects the active form of folate, methyltetrahydrofolic acid, from oxidation. Thus, the bioavailability of folate increases in your body, and you get enhanced health benefits from it.

VITAMIN C AND IRON

Iron is important in hemoglobin formation and the production of healthy red blood cells. Vitamin C Increases your body's absorption of iron, so taking iron with vitamin C makes more iron available for RBC production than taking iron alone. Eat iron-rich foods such as spinach, lentils, and beans with vitamin C-rich foods such as bell peppers, Indian gooseberries, and lemons.

VITAMIN C AND ZINC

Vitamin C and zinc have a synergistic relationship. Both have antioxidant properties and both are important for immune function. Eating vitamin C-rich foods like citrus fruits, bell peppers and zinc-rich foods such as chickpeas, pumpkin seeds and lentils together can synergistically boost your immune defense.

FOLATE AND VITAMIN B12

Taking naturally sourced folate along with vitamin B12 produces a synergistic effect. These two vitamins work together to help iron function better in your body. Vitamin B9 works together with vitamin B12 in the production of red blood cells. They work together to produce a compound, S-adenosylmethionine (SAMe), that is involved in boosting your mood and immune function and relieving pain associated with osteoarthritis. It also helps prevent depression and liver diseases.

VITAMIN B6, VITAMIN B9 AND VITAMIN B12

Eating foods rich in vitamins B6, B9, and B12 together can significantly lower your homocysteine levels, which can help lower your risk of stroke and cardiovascular disease. Vitamin B6, folate, and vitamin B12 are all involved in the metabolism of homocysteine. Vitamin B6 is involved in converting the amino acid homocysteine to cysteine, while folate and vitamin B12 are involved in converting homocysteine back to methionine.

VITAMIN B2 AND VITAMIN B9

Riboflavin, or vitamin B2, enhances the activity of folate. Vitamin B9 or folate has an important metabolic interaction with riboflavin. Folate requires riboflavin to effectively form methionine from homocysteine. The riboflavin derivative flavin adenine dinucleotide (FAD) acts as a coenzyme for 5,10-methylenetetrahydrofolate reductase (MTHFR), which is a folate-metabolizing enzyme. FAD-dependent MTHFR catalyzes the reaction that yields the active form of folate, 5-methyltetrahydrofolate, which is needed to form methionine from homocysteine.

POTENTIALLY DANGEROUS VITAMIN COMBINATIONS YOU SHOULD AVOID

VITAMIN C AND VITAMIN B12

Taking vitamin C with foods containing vitamin B12 affects the absorption of vitamin B12 in your body, and you do not get the health benefits of vitamin B12. Vitamin C can partially inactivate hydroxycobalamin as well as the intrinsic factor, which is necessary for the absorption of vitamin B12. Keep a gap of at least two hours between the intake of vitamin C and vitamin B12.

VITAMIN B12 AND BAKING SODA

Vitamin B12 is bound to protein in food. Gastric acid is needed to break this vitamin B12-protein bond and release free vitamin B12. Baking soda works primarily by neutralizing the acid in your stomach. Low stomach acidity causes vitamin B12 to remain in the bound form and pass out of your body without being absorbed, even if your vitamin B12 consumption is high.

FOLIC ACID AND VITAMIN B12

Folate from natural foods works positively with vitamin B12 to form healthy red blood cells. However, taking folic acid through dietary supplements with vitamin B12 can be harmful. High doses of folic acid, more than 1mg or 1,000 mcg, can mask a vitamin B12 deficiency. You may not even know that you are deficient in Vitamin B12, which can delay treatment and increase your risk of depression, fatigue, hair and skin problems.

WATER-SOLUBLE AND FAT-SOLUBLE VITAMINS

It is not advised to take water-soluble vitamins (B and C) with fat-soluble vitamins (A, D, E, and K) because they are absorbed differently in the body. Mixing them may reduce the health benefits you get from each of them. Water-soluble vitamins are more absorbed on an empty stomach (except for vitamin B12, which is well absorbed with food), while fat-soluble vitamins require the presence of fat in your body to be absorbed. To maximize the benefits of each type of vitamin, eat foods rich in B and C in the morning and foods rich in A, D, E, and K in the evening. If you are taking vitamin supplements, take B and C on an empty stomach and take fat-soluble vitamins in the evening after a meal.

UNIT 5
DIET PLAN

Here's a weekly diet plan to include natural sources rich in vitamins B1, B2, B3, B5, B6, B7, B9, B12 and vitamin C in your diet. Repeat this diet plan every seven days, and you will never be deficient in water-soluble vitamins.

VITAMIN B1

Day 1: Two slices of whole wheat bread and one cup of milk.

Day 2: One cup of brown rice with mixed dal (lentils)

Day 3: One cup of boiled green peas + A handful of roasted pistachios.

Day 4: A bowl of oatmeal with milk + one tablespoon flaxseeds.

Day 5: A handful of roasted sunflower seeds + one cup of cooked soybeans with chapatti.

Day 6: Two slices of whole wheat bread with lentil soup.

Day 7: One cup of baked acorn squash with herbed brown rice.

VITAMIN B2

Day 1: One cup of almond milk shake.

Day 2: One cup of cooked spinach with a bowl of quinoa + a handful of almonds.

Day 3: One cup of grilled mushrooms + one cup of cooked soybeans and kidney beans.

Day 4: One cup curd + one avocado + a handful of almonds.

Day 5: Mushroom and beans pot pie with cheese toppings.

Day 6: One cup of milk + one cup of dark green leafy vegetable with brown rice.

Day 7: A bowl of yogurt fruit salad + a bowl of cooked quinoa.

VITAMIN B3

Day 1: A handful of roasted peanuts.

Day 2: One cup of grilled mushrooms seasoned with sesame seeds + A bowl of brown rice.

Day 3: Whole wheat chapatti with mushroom masala + a handful of sunflower seeds.

Day 4: Mixed dal with brown rice + a large mango.

Day 5: A cup of cooked green peas + a handful of peanuts + A bowl of whole grain of your choice + one avocado.

Day 6: A bowl of beans + a potato dish with added tahini + brown rice.

Day 7: Baked sweet potato with peas and beans + a handful of peanuts.

VITAMIN B5

Day 1: One cup of grilled shiitake mushrooms.

Day 2: A handful of roasted sunflower seeds + one large avocado.

Day 3: One and a half cups of cooked broccoli with peanuts + oatmeal with milk.

Day 4: Mashed potato + One cup of chopped watermelon + a handful of sunflower seeds.

Day 5: One cup of cooked chickpeas + a bowl of yogurt fruit salad + a handful of peanuts + one avocado.

Day 6: Mushroom soup + potato dish + a handful of peanuts.

Day 7: Milk with multigrain bread + Frankie with chickpeas fillings.

VITAMIN B6

Day 1: One bowl of cooked chickpeas with brown rice + a handful of sunflower seeds.

Day 2: Soybean gravy with whole wheat chapatti + one large mango + a handful of mixed nuts.

Day 3: A bowl of bulgur/daliya + banana milkshake + sweet potato dish.

Day 4: One cup of cooked soybeans with brown rice + one avocado + a handful of mixed nuts.

Day 5: One large baked sweet potato + a bowl of bulger + one large mango.

Day 6: A handful of sunflower seeds + brown rice with beans + one banana.

Day 7: Roasted chickpeas + carrot dish + a handful of pistachios.

VITAMIN B7

Day 1: Mushroom soup + a handful of walnuts + a cup of coffee.

Day 2: One baked sweet potato + a handful of peanuts + a cup of grilled mushrooms.

Day 3: One cup of cooked soybean + a handful of walnuts.

Day 4: A small bowl of amaranth grain salad.

Day 5: One cup grilled portabella mushrooms + soybean dish.

Day 6: A cup of cooked kidney beans with naan made from amaranth flour and whole wheat flour + a handful of sunflower seeds.

Day 7: Soybean gravy + a handful of peanuts + a cup of coffee + strawberries.

VITAMIN B9

Day 1: One cup of cooked spinach with soybean and black-eye peas.

Day 2: Four spears of steamed asparagus + one cup of cooked broccoli + a handful of sunflower seeds + one beetroot.

Day 3: One and a half cups of steamed Brussels sprouts, cauliflower, and broccoli + + one small papaya fruit + a handful of peanuts.

Day 4: Half a cup of cooked mixed leafy greens + tomato salad + one avocado.

Day 5: ¾ cup of cooked kidney beans in tomato gravy + one large avocado + a handful of mixed nuts.

Day 6: One cup of cooked Brussels sprouts + one cup of black eye peas + beetroot and tomato salad + one boiled sweet corn.

Day 7: One cup of cooked green soybeans+ sweet corn soup + one large beetroot + one orange.

VITAMIN B12

Day 1: One cup of milk + a bowl of mushroom with cheese + a bowl of yogurt fruit salad.

Day 2: One bowl of yogurt + paneer tikka (cottage cheese tikka) + one banana + one cup of milk.

Day 3: Yogurt dishes like *kadhi* + Any homemade sweet made from milk (burfi, halwa, milk cake) + flavored milkshake.

Day 4: Sourdough bread with cheese + one scope vanilla ice cream + a bowl of *raita* + an apple.

Day 5: A glass of buttermilk + *uttapam* made with fermented batter + half a cup of chopped watermelons + a cup of milk.

Day 6: One cup of yogurt + fermented dishes like *dhokla* and *khaman* + one orange + a cup of banana milk.

Day 7: One cup banana milk + mushroom paneer sabzi with chapatti (dough kneaded using whey liquid of cottage cheese) + a bowl of cucumber *raita*

VITAMIN C

Day 1: Two oranges.

Day 2: One cup of sliced strawberries.

Day 3: One cup of fresh papaya chunks.

Day 4: One and a half cups steamed broccoli.

Day 5: One and a half green kiwi or one gold kiwi.

Day 6: handful of blackcurrants.

Day 7: One guava.

Eat So What! The Science of Water-Soluble Vitamins.....La Fonceur

UNIT 6
RECIPES

Cup size used in recipes: 200 g

SOYBEAN SALAD

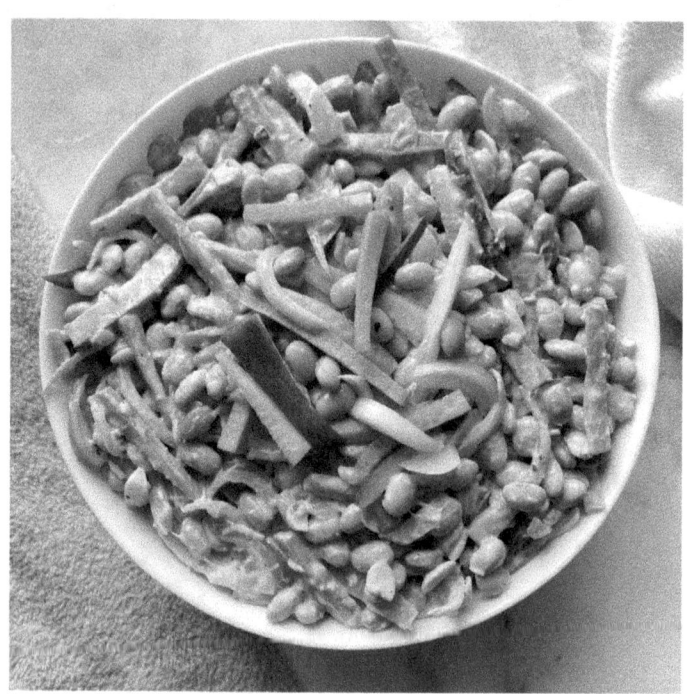

Ingredients

Dry soybeans: 125 g	Onion: 1
Cucumber: 1	Carrot: 1
Black pepper powder: ½ tsp.	Apple cider vinegar: 1 tbsp.
Powdered sugar: 1 tbsp.	Salt: to taste
Hung curd: 3 tbsp	Water: 2 cups

Method

1. Soak soybeans in water overnight for 8 hours.

2. Wash soybeans well and cook with salt and water for 2 whistles or till tender. Turn off the flame. Drain the water.

3. Meanwhile, cut onion, carrot and cucumber lengthwise. Add salt over the veggies. Mix and keep covered for 15 minutes. The veggies will release water. Drain the water.

4. Take all the veggies and soybeans in a bowl. Add hung curd, apple cider vinegar, salt, black pepper and sugar. Mix well.

5. Chill the salad in the refrigerator for half an hour and serve.

VEGETABLE PANEER TIKKA

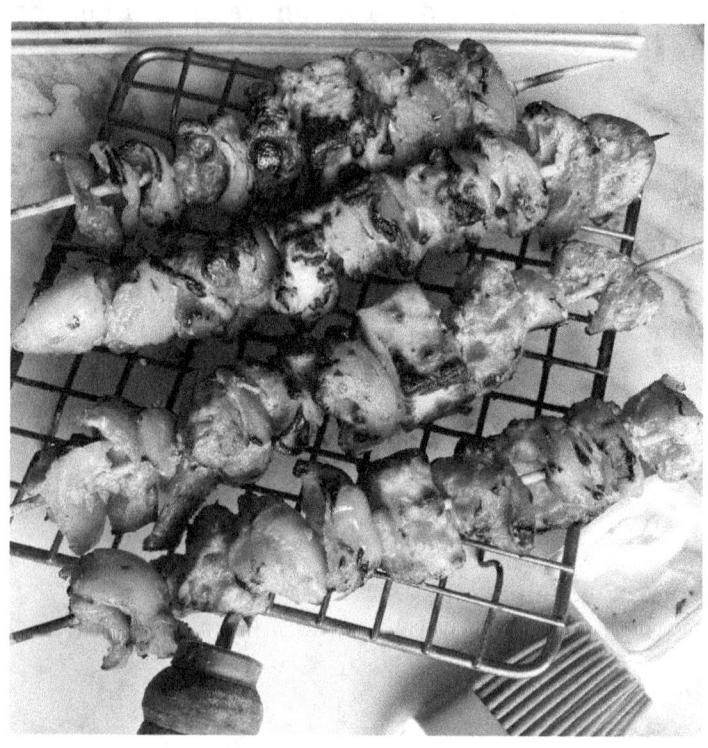

Ingredients

Hung curd: 250 g	Cottage cheese: 200 g
Yellow bell pepper: 1	Red bell pepper: 1
Green bell pepper: 1	Tomatoes: 2
Mushrooms: 200 g	Onions: 3

Roasted chickpea flour (besan): 3 tbsp.	Turmeric powder: ½ tsp.
Coriander leaves: 1 cup	Mint leaves: ¾ cup
Ginger: 1 ½ inch	Garlic: 12-15 cloves
Garam masala: 1 tsp.	Mustard oil: 2 tbsp.
Lemon juice: 1 tbsp.	Black salt: ½ tsp.
Salt: to taste	Butter: 10 g
Barbecue stick skewers:	10-12

Method

1. Take coriander leaves, mint leaves, ginger, lemon juice, and black salt in a mixer jar. Add 2 tbsp. of hung curd and grind well.

2. Cut all the vegetables and cottage cheese into 1-inch cubes. Add coriander chutney, vegetables, chopped garlic, turmeric powder, garam masala, mustard oil, salt, and roasted gram flour to the hung curd and mix well. Cover and refrigerate for 4 hours to marinate.

3. The vegetables will release water and discard the liquid. Arrange each vegetable and cottage cheese on bamboo skewers.

4. Place a metal rack over a direct flame and place two to three sticks at a time. Cook on all sides. Alternatively, grill tikka using the grill function of your oven or in a griller.

5. Once done, apply butter and enjoy the vegetable paneer tikka.

MASALA UTTAPAM

Ingredients

For Uttapam batter

Split black lentils: 1 cup	Parboiled rice: 3 cups
Fenugreek seeds: ½ tsp.	Sugar: 1 tsp.
Salt: To taste	Water: ½ cup

For Uttapam masala

Onion: 1	Green peas: ½ cup
Chopped carrots: ½ cup	Split black lentils: 1 tbsp.
Split Bengal gram: 1 tbsp.	Mustard seeds: 1 tsp.
Curry leaves: 12	Asafetida: A pinch
Sambhar masala: 1 ½ tbsp.	Turmeric powder: ½ tsp.
Green chillies: 2	Oil: To make uttapam

Method

1. Take parboiled rice (use regular rice if parboiled rice is not available), split black lentils, and fenugreek seeds in a bowl. Wash them well. Add water to it. Cover and leave for 4-5 hours.

2. Drain the water and grind them coarsely in a grinder with ½ cup water. The batter should be thin enough to be poured but not too runny.

3. Add sugar and keep the batter in a warm place for 12 hours, preferably in an oven. It may take up to 20 hours, depending on the weather conditions.

4. Once fermented, you will see bubbles, and the batter will rise. Add salt.

5. Heat oil in a pan. Add mustard seeds to it. Add asafetida, curry leaves, split black lentils, and Bengal gram when they crackle. Cook for two minutes.

6. Add onion and green chilies. Cook for 5 minutes.

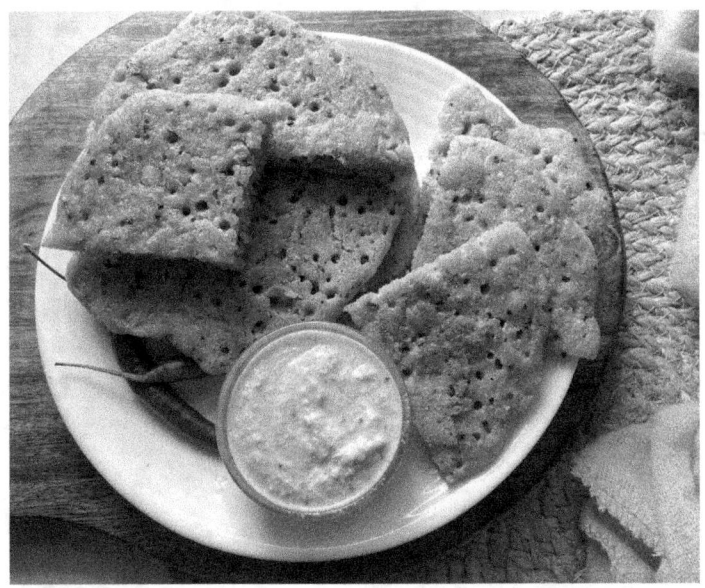

7. Add green peas, chopped carrots and salt. Cover and cook for 5 minutes.

8. Add turmeric powder and sambhar masala (use garam masala if you do not have sambhar masala) and

mix well. Cover and cook for 5-7 minutes, and turn off the flame. Mix the prepared masala with the uttapam batter.

9. Pour a spoon of oil on a hot pan. Pour a ladle of the masala uttapam batter and spread it like a pancake. Cover and cook for 3-4 minutes.

10. Apply a little oil on the top and sides of the surface. Flip the uttapam and cook for 2 minutes on the other side as well. Serve it with peanut chutney.

PEANUT CHUTNEY

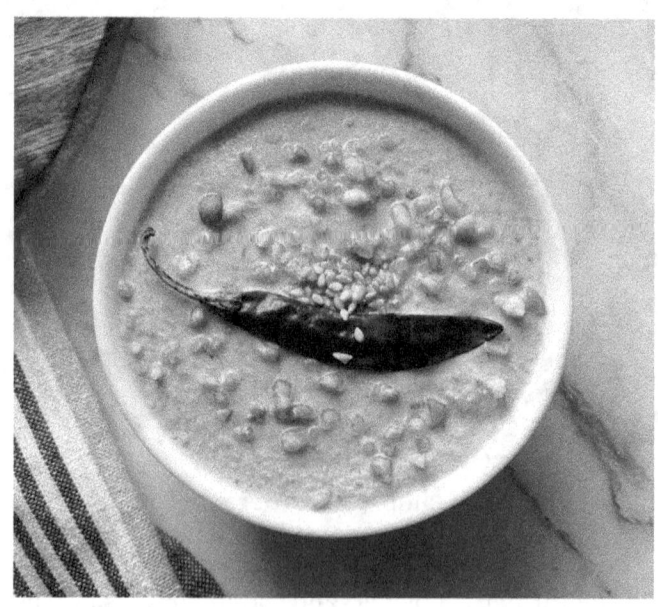

Ingredients

Peanuts: 1 cup (110 g)	Sesame seeds: 1 tbsp.
Split black lentils: 1 tbsp.	Red chilies: 2 (seedless)
Garlic: 4 cloves	Curry leaves: 12
Cumin seeds: 1 tsp.	Lemon juice: 1 tbsp.
Salt: To taste	Water: ½ cup

Method

1. Dry roast the peanuts. Once cooled, rub them in a kitchen towel and peel off the skin.

2. Dry roast sesame seeds and lentils separately.

3. Put all the ingredients in a mixer jar and grind by adding water as required. Adjust the amount of water as per taste. Serve with uttapam.

MIXED DAL

Ingredients

Yellow split pigeon peas: 4 tbsp.

Split black lentils: 2 tbsp.

Split green gram (moong dal): 2 tbsp.

Bengal gram (split): 2 tbsp.

Red lentils: 2 tbsp.

Turmeric powder: ½ tsp.

Salt: To taste

Water: 600 ml

For tempering

Asafetida: A pinch

Dry red chillies: 2

Cloves: 3

Bay leaf: 1

Cinnamon: 1 inch

Cumin seeds: 1 tsp.

Curry leaves: 12

Garlic: 8-10 cloves

Garam masala: 1 tsp.

Coriander-cumin powder: 1 tsp.

Ghee: 1 ½ tbsp.

Water: 200 ml

Method

1. Wash the lentils and soak them in enough water for 15 minutes. Wash the lentils thoroughly and drain.

2. Put the lentils in a pressure cooker and add 600 ml water, turmeric powder, and salt. Bring to a boil. Remove the foam from the top of the dal. Close the lid and cook for 2 whistles or until cooked.

3. Heat ghee in a pan. Add chopped red chilies, cloves, bay leaf, cinnamon, cumin seeds, curry leaves and asafetida. Cook for 2 minutes.

4. Add chopped garlic and cook until light brown.

5. Add garam masala and coriander cumin powder. Cook for a minute. Add the dal and mix well. Add 200 ml water and turn the flame to high.

6. Cook for 5 minutes until the dal thickens slightly. Turn off the flame and serve with herbed rice.

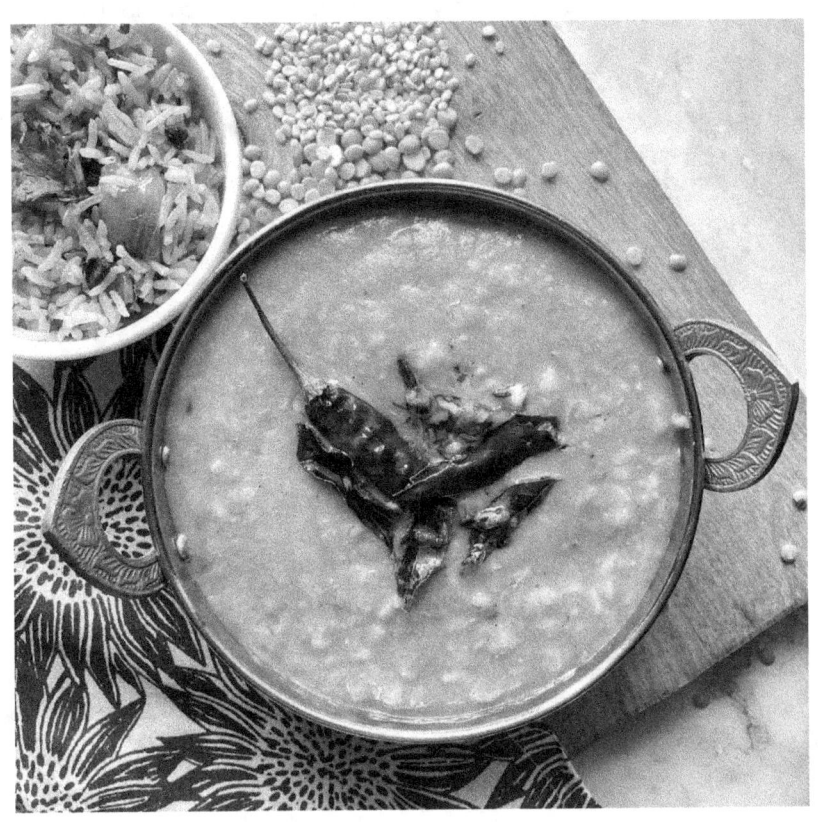

HERBED BROWN RICE

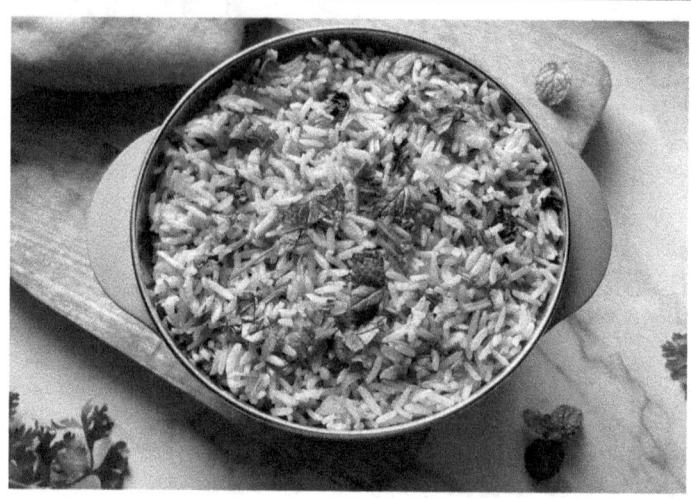

Ingredients

Cooked brown rice: 2 cups	Garlic: 6 cloves
Onion: 1 medium	Indian basil leaves: 15
Mint leaves: 15	Coriander leaves: 50 g
Salt: To taste	Ghee/Butter: 1 tbsp.

Method

1. Chop basil, mint and coriander leaves.

2. Heat ghee in a pan. Add garlic and cook for 2-3 minutes. Add onion and salt. Cook for 5 minutes.

3. Add chopped herbs and cook for a minute. Add brown rice and mix well. Cook for 5 minutes. Serve hot with mixed dal.

NUTTY COLD COFFEE

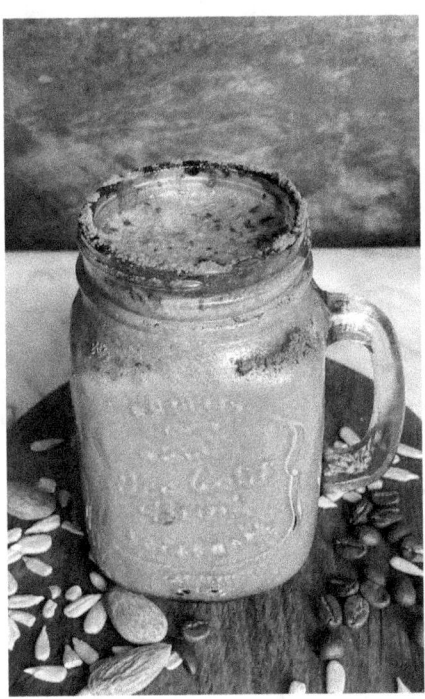

Ingredients

Oats: ½ cup
Milk: 600 ml
Almonds: 15
Walnuts: 3 kernels
Sunflower seeds: 1 tbsp.
Coffee: 2 tbsp
Cocoa powder: 2 tbsp.
Honey: 2 tbsp. + as required
Water: 1½ cups
Ice: 5-6

Method

1. Cook the oats in water for 5 minutes till mushy. Let it cool to room temperature.

2. Add all the ingredients except the nuts in a blender and blend till smooth.

3. Add the almonds, walnuts, and sunflower seeds and blend again. Serve chilled.

READ PREVIOUS BOOKS OF THE EAT SO WHAT! SERIES

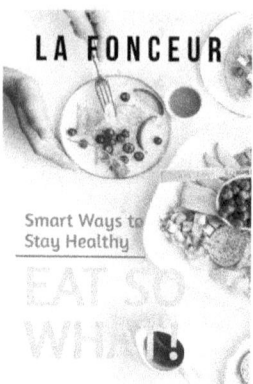

Book 1:

Eat So What! Smart Ways to Stay Healthy

Book 2:

Eat So What! The Power of Vegetarianism

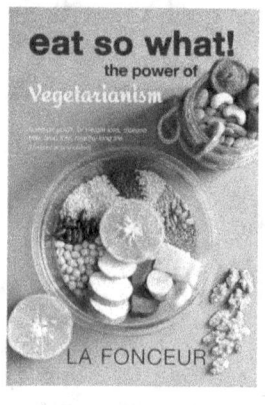

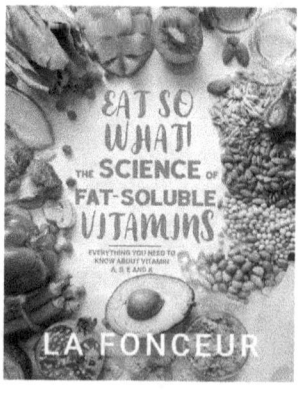

Book 3:

Eat So What! The Science of Fat-Soluble Vitamins

REFERENCES

1. Fonceur L. Basics of Vitamins. Eat So What! The Science of Fat-Soluble Vitamin. Oct 2023.
2. Clements RS Jr, Darnell B. Myo-inositol content of common foods: development of a high-myo-inositol diet. Am J Clin Nutr. 1980 Sep;33(9):1954-67. doi: 10.1093/ajcn/33.9.1954. PMID: 7416064.
3. Pepe S, Rosenfeldt F. Tissue Ageing: From Molecular Mechanisms to Clinical Perspectives. Experimental Gerontology, 2008.
4. Tamer CE, Sinir GO. Amygdalin. Non-Alcoholic Beverages, 2019
5. Laetrile (amygdalin or vitamin B17). Cancer Research UK.
6. Fonceur L. Not True Vitamins but Still Vitamins! Eat So What! The Science of Fat-Soluble Vitamins. 2023 Sep. Page 13-15.
7. Thiamin Deficiency (Beriberi; Vitamin B1 Deficiency) By Larry E. Johnson, MSD Manual Professional version.
8. Thornalley PJ. The potential role of thiamine (vitamin B1) in diabetic complications. Curr Diabetes Rev. 2005 Aug;1(3):287-98. doi: 10.2174/157339905774574383. PMID: 18220605.
9. Richard H. Thiamine Deficiency and Diabetic Polyneuropathy Compelling evidence for an interrelationship. Natural Medicine Journal. 2018 Nov 7.
10. Mrowicka M, Mrowicki J, Dragan G, Majsterek I. The importance of thiamine (vitamin B1) in humans. Biosci Rep. 2023 Oct 31;43(10):BSR20230374. doi: 10.1042/BSR20230374. PMID: 37389565; PMCID: PMC10568373.
11. Małgorzata Mrowicka, Jerzy Mrowicki, Grzegorz Dragan, Ireneusz Majsterek; The importance of thiamine (vitamin B1) in humans. Biosci Rep Oct 31 2023; 43 (10): BSR20230374. doi: https://doi.org/10.1042/BSR20230374
12. Menezes R, Godin A, Rodrigues FF. Thiamine and riboflavin inhibit production of cytokines and increase the anti-inflammatory activity of a corticosteroid in a chronic model of inflammation induced by complete Freund's adjuvant. Pharmacological Reports, Volume 69, Issue 5, 2017, Pages 1036-1043, ISSN 1734-1140, https://doi.org/10.1016/j.pharep.2017.04.011.
13. Zaringhalam J, Akbari A, Zali A, Manaheji H, Nazemian V, Shadnoush M, Ezzatpanah S. Long-Term Treatment by Vitamin B1 and Reduction of Serum Proinflammatory Cytokines, Hyperalgesia, and Paw Edema in Adjuvant-Induced Arthritis. Basic Clin Neurosci. 2016 Oct;7(4):331-340. doi: 10.15412/J.BCN.03070406. PMID: 27872694; PMCID: PMC5102562.

14. Helali J, Park S, Ziaeian B, Han JK, Lankarani-Fard A. Thiamine and Heart Failure: Challenging Cases of Modern-Day Cardiac Beriberi. Mayo Clin Proc Innov Qual Outcomes. 2019 May 27;3(2):221-225. doi: 10.1016/j.mayocpiqo.2019.03.003. PMID: 31193878; PMCID: PMC6543258.
15. Baltrusch S. The Role of Neurotropic B Vitamins in Nerve Regeneration. Biomed Res Int. 2021 Jul 13;2021:9968228. doi: 10.1155/2021/9968228. PMID: 34337067; PMCID: PMC8294980.
16. Bakker SJ, Leunissen KM. Hypothesis on cellular ATP depletion and adenosine release as causes of heart failure and vasodilatation in cardiovascular beriberi. Med Hypotheses. 1995 Sep;45(3):265-7. doi: 10.1016/0306-9877(95)90115-9. PMID: 8569549.
17. Beltramo E, Mazzeo A, Porta M. Thiamine and diabetes: back to the future? Acta Diabetol. 2021 Nov;58(11):1433-1439. doi: 10.1007/s00592-021-01752-4. Epub 2021 Jun 5. PMID: 34091762; PMCID: PMC8505293.
18. Bakker S, Low thiamine intake and risk of cataract, Ophthalmology, Elsevier, July 2001
19. Leavening agents, yeast, baker's, active dry – Food Data Central. US Department of Agriculture.
20. Riboflavin Fact Sheet for Health Professionals. National Institute of Health. Office of Dietary Supplements
21. Riboflavin Deficiency (Vitamin B2 Deficiency) By Larry E. Johnson, MSD Professional version.
22. Mahabadi N, Bhusal A, Banks SW. Riboflavin Deficiency. [Updated 2023 Jul 17]. In: StatPearls [Internet]. Treasure Island (FL): StatPearls Publishing; 2024 Jan-. Available from: https://www.ncbi.nlm.nih.gov/books/NBK470460/
23. Aljaadi AM, Devlin AM, Green TJ. Riboflavin intake and status and relationship to anemia. Nutr Rev. 2022 Dec 6;81(1):114-132. doi: 10.1093/nutrit/nuac043. PMID: 36018769.
24. Udhayabanu T, Manole A, Rajeshwari M, Varalakshmi P, Houlden H, Ashokkumar B. Riboflavin Responsive Mitochondrial Dysfunction in Neurodegenerative Diseases. J Clin Med. 2017 May 5;6(5):52. doi: 10.3390/jcm6050052. PMID: 28475111; PMCID: PMC5447943.
25. Szczuko M, Ziętek M, Kulpa D, Seidler T. Riboflavin - properties, occurrence and its use in medicine. De Gruyter. Pteridines 2019; 30: 33–47 https://doi.org/10.1515/pteridines-2019-0004.
26. Namazi N, Heshmati J, Tarighat-Esfanjani A. Supplementation with Riboflavin (Vitamin B2) for Migraine Prophylaxis in Adults and Children: A Review. Int J Vitam Nutr Res. 2015;85(1-2):79-87. doi: 10.1024/0300-9831/a000225. PMID: 26780280.
27. Cosimo Mazzotta, Stefano Caragiuli, Aldo Caporossi, Chapter 13 - Riboflavin and the Cornea and Implications for Cataracts.

Handbook of Nutrition, Diet and the Eye, Academic Press, 2014, Pages 123-130, https://doi.org/10.1016/B978-0-12-401717-7.00013-7.

28. Shane B. Folate and vitamin B12 metabolism: overview and interaction with riboflavin, vitamin B6, and polymorphisms. Food Nutr Bull. 2008 Jun;29(2 Suppl):S5-16; discussion S17-9. doi: 10.1177/15648265080292S103. PMID: 18709878.

29. Ued FV, Mathias MG, Toffano RBD, et al. Vitamin B2 and Folate Concentrations are Associated with ARA, EPA and DHA Fatty Acids in Red Blood Cells of Brazilian Children and Adolescents. Nutrients. 2019;11(12):2918. Published 2019 Dec 2. doi:10.3390/nu11122918 Fratoni V, Brandi ML. B vitamins, homocysteine and bone health. Nutrients. 2015 Mar 30;7(4):2176-92. doi: 10.3390/nu7042176. PMID: 25830943; PMCID: PMC4425139.

30. Cimino JA, Jhangiani S, Schwartz E, Cooperman JM. Riboflavin metabolism in the hypothyroid human adult. Proc Soc Exp Biol Med. 1987 Feb;184(2):151-3. doi: 10.3181/00379727-184-42459. PMID: 3809170.

31. Parkington DA, Koulman A, and Jones K S. Protocol for measuring erythrocyte glutathione reductase activity coefficient to assess riboflavin status. Nov 24, 2023. Star Protocols. DOI: 10.1016/j.xpro.2023.102726.

32. Moat SJ, Ashfield-Watt PA, Powers HJ, Newcombe RG, McDowell IF. Effect of riboflavin status on the homocysteine-lowering effect of folate in relation to the MTHFR (C677T) genotype. Clin Chem. 2003 Feb;49(2):295-302. doi: 10.1373/49.2.295. PMID: 12560354.

33. Blom HJ, Smulders Y. Overview of homocysteine and folate metabolism. With special references to cardiovascular disease and neural tube defects. J Inherit Metab Dis. 2011 Feb;34(1):75-81. doi: 10.1007/s10545-010-9177-4. Epub 2010 Sep 4. PMID: 20814827; PMCID: PMC3026708.

34. Olfat N, Ashoori M, Saedisomeolia A. Riboflavin is an antioxidant: a review update. Br J Nutr. 2022 Nov 28;128(10):1887-1895. doi: 10.1017/S0007114521005031. Epub 2022 Feb 4. PMID: 35115064.

35. Zhang H, Forman HJ. Glutathione synthesis and its role in redox signaling. Semin Cell Dev Biol. 2012 Sep;23(7):722-8. doi: 10.1016/j.semcdb.2012.03.017. Epub 2012 Apr 3. PMID: 22504020; PMCID: PMC3422610.

36. Mazzotta, Cosimo & Caragiuli, Stefano & Caporossi, Aldo. (2014). Riboflavin and the Cornea and Implications for Cataracts. 10.1016/B978-0-12-401717-7.00013-7.

37. Food Data Central, US Department of Agriculture. Mushrooms, White, Raw (Sr Legacy, 169251) Mushrooms, White, Raw.

38. Food Data Central, US Department of Agriculture. Seeds, Sunflower Seeds.
39. Niacin: Fact Sheet for Health Professionals. National Institutes of Health. Office of Dietary Supplements
40. Hopp AK, Grüter P, Hottiger MO. Regulation of Glucose Metabolism by NAD+ and ADP-Ribosylation. Cells. 2019 Aug 13;8(8):890. doi: 10.3390/cells8080890. Erratum in: Cells. 2019 Oct 31;8(11):E1371. doi: 10.3390/cells8111371. PMID: 31412683; PMCID: PMC6721828.
41. Cooper GM. The Cell: A Molecular Approach. 2nd edition. Sunderland (MA): Sinauer Associates; 2000. The Mechanism of Oxidative Phosphorylation.
42. C. Robin Ganellin. Discovery of the cholesterol absorption inhibitor, ezetimibe. Introduction to Biological and Small Molecule Drug Research and Development, 2013.
43. Hrubša M, Siatka T, Nejmanová I, Mladěnka P. On Behalf of The Oemonom. Biological Properties of Vitamins of the B-Complex, Part 1: Vitamins B1, B2, B3, and B5. Nutrients. 2022 Jan 22;14(3):484. doi: 10.3390/nu14030484. PMID: 35276844; PMCID: PMC8839250.
44. Heintze T, Wilhelm D, Schmidlin T, Klein K. Effects of Diminished NADPH:cytochrome P450 Reductase in Human Hepatocytes on Lipid and Bile Acid Homeostasis. Front Pharmacol. 2021 Nov 15;12:769703. doi: 10.3389/fphar.2021.769703. PMID: 34867397; PMCID: PMC8634102.
45. Schiffer L, Barnard L, Baranowski ES, Gilligan LC, Taylor AE, Arlt W, Shackleton CHL, Storbeck KH. Human steroid biosynthesis, metabolism and excretion are differentially reflected by serum and urine steroid metabolomes: A comprehensive review. J Steroid Biochem Mol Biol. 2019 Nov;194:105439. doi: 10.1016/j.jsbmb.2019.105439. Epub 2019 Jul 27. PMID: 31362062; PMCID: PMC6857441.
46. J.P. Kamat & T.P.A. Devasagayam (1999) Nicotinamide (vitamin B3) as an effective antioxidant against oxidative damage in rat brain mitochondria, Redox Report, 4:4, 179-184, DOI: 10.1179/135100099101534882.
47. Lu J, Holmgren A. The thioredoxin antioxidant system. Free Radical Biology and Medicine. Volume 66, 2014, Pages 75-87. https://doi.org/10.1016/j.freeradbiomed.2013.07.036.
48. Pan J, Zhou Y, Pang N, Yang L. Dietary Niacin Intake and Mortality Among Individuals With Nonalcoholic Fatty Liver Disease. JAMA Network Open. 2024;7(2):e2354277. doi:10.1001/jamanetworkopen.2023.54277.
49. Villanueva M. DNA Damage, DNA Repair, and Micronutrients in Aging. Molecular Basis of Nutrition and Aging, 2016.

50. Soudijn W, van Wijngaarden I, Ijzerman AP. Nicotinic acid receptor subtypes and their ligands. Med Res Rev. 2007 May;27(3):417-33. doi: 10.1002/med.20102. PMID: 17238156.
51. Agledal L, Niere M & Ziegler M. The phosphate makes a difference: cellular functions of NADP, Redox Report, 15:1, 2-10, 2010. DOI: 10.1179/174329210X12650506623122.
52. Cholesterol Medicines Guide from the FDA Office of Women's Health.
53. Kamanna, VS, Kashyap M. Mechanism of Action of Niacin. American Journal of Cardiology, Volume 101, Issue 8, S20 - S26.
54. Kashyap ML, Ganji S, Nakra NK, Kamanna VS. Niacin for treatment of nonalcoholic fatty liver disease (NAFLD): novel use for an old drug? J Clin Lipidol. 2019 Nov-Dec;13(6):873-879. doi: 10.1016/j.jacl.2019.10.006. Epub 2019 Oct 14. PMID: 31706905.
55. Jonas, W.B., Rapoza, C.P. & Blair, W.F. The effect of niacinamide on osteoarthritis: A pilot study. Inflamm Res 45, 330–334 (1996). https://doi.org/10.1007/BF02252945.
56. Swerdlow RH. Is NADH effective in the treatment of Parkinson's disease? Drugs Aging. 1998 Oct;13(4):263-8. doi: 10.2165/00002512-199813040-00002. PMID: 9805207.
57. Gasperi V, Sibilano M, Savini I, Catani MV. Niacin in the Central Nervous System: An Update of Biological Aspects and Clinical Applications. Int J Mol Sci. 2019 Feb 23;20(4):974. doi: 10.3390/ijms20040974. PMID: 30813414; PMCID: PMC6412771.
58. Domanico D, Verboschi F, Altimari S, Zompatori L, Vingolo EM. Ocular Effects of Niacin: A Review of the Literature. Med Hypothesis Discov Innov Ophthalmol. 2015 Summer;4(2):64-71. PMID: 26060832; PMCID: PMC4458328.
59. Hou, J., Wen, Y., Gao, S. et al. Association of dietary intake of B vitamins with glaucoma. Sci Rep 14, 8539 (2024). https://doi.org/10.1038/s41598-024-58526-5.
60. Food Data Central, US Department of Agriculture. Potatoes, Gold, Without Skin, Raw (Foundation, 2346403).
61. Food Data Central, US Department of Agriculture. Sweet Potato, Cooked, Baked in Skin, Flesh, Without Salt (Sr Legacy, 168483).
62. Food Data Central, US Department of Agriculture. Mangos, Raw (Sr Legacy, 169910).
63. Pantothenic Acid - Fact Sheet for Health Professionals. National Institutes of Health - Office of Dietary Supplements.
64. Aprahamian M, Dentinger A, Stock-Damgé C, Kouassi JC, Grenier JF. Effects of supplemental pantothenic acid on wound healing: experimental study in rabbit. Am J Clin Nutr. 1985 Mar;41(3):578-89. doi: 10.1093/ajcn/41.3.578. PMID: 3976557.

65. Gheita AA, Gheita TA, Kenawy SA. The potential role of B5: A stitch in time and switch in cytokine. Phytotherapy Research. 2020; 34: 306–314. https://doi.org/10.1002/ptr.6537

66. Sanvictores T, Chauhan S. Vitamin B5 (Pantothenic Acid) [Updated 2024 Feb 29]. In: StatPearls [Internet]. Treasure Island (FL): StatPearls Publishing; 2024 Jan-. Available from: https://www.ncbi.nlm.nih.gov/books/NBK563233/

67. He W, Hu S, Du X, Wen Q, Zhong XP, Zhou X, Zhou C, Xiong W, Gao Y, Zhang S, Wang R, Yang J, Ma L. Vitamin B5 Reduces Bacterial Growth via Regulating Innate Immunity and Adaptive Immunity in Mice Infected with Mycobacterium tuberculosis. Front Immunol. 2018 Feb 26;9:365. doi: 10.3389/fimmu.2018.00365. PMID: 29535733; PMCID: PMC5834509.

68. Huisjes R, Card DJ. Methods for assessment of pantothenic acid (Vitamin B5). Laboratory Assessment of Vitamin Status, 2019.

69. Sanvictores T, Chauhan S. Vitamin B5 (Pantothenic Acid) [Updated 2024 Feb 29]. Treasure Island (FL): StatPearls Publishing.

70. Michael T, Murray ND, John Nowicki ND. Pantethine. Textbook of Natural Medicine (Fifth Edition), 2020.

71. Rucker RB, Pantothenic Acid. Encyclopedia of Food and Health, 2016.

72. Aprahamian M, Dentinger A, Stock-Damgé C, Kouassi JC, Grenier JF. Effects of supplemental pantothenic acid on wound healing: experimental study in rabbit. Am J Clin Nutr. 1985 Mar;41(3):578-89. doi: 10.1093/ajcn/41.3.578. PMID: 3976557.

73. Weimann BI, Hermann D. Studies on wound healing: effects of calcium D-pantothenate on the migration, proliferation and protein synthesis of human dermal fibroblasts in culture. Int J Vitam Nutr Res. 1999 Mar;69(2):113-9. doi: 10.1024/0300-9831.69.2.113. PMID: 10218148.

74. Casas C. Vitamins.Analysis of Cosmetic Products, 2007.

75. Shi J, Wang L, Zhang Y, Zhi D. Clinical efficacy of vitamin B in the treatment of mouth ulcer: a systematic review and meta-analysis. Annals of Palliative Medicine, North America, 10, Jun. 2021.

76. Xu J, Patassini S, Begley P, Garth JS. Cerebral deficiency of vitamin B5 (d-pantothenic acid; pantothenate) as a potentially-reversible cause of neurodegeneration and dementia in sporadic Alzheimer's disease. Biochemical and Biophysical Research Communications. Volume 527, Issue 3, 2020. Pages 676-681. ISSN 0006-291X. https://doi.org/10.1016/j.bbrc.2020.05.015.

77. Fooddata Central - US Department of Agriculture. Wheat Flour, Whole-Grain (Includes Foods For Usda's Food Distribution Program) (Sr Legacy, 168893).

78. Vitamin B6 fact sheet for health professionals. National Institutes of Health – Office of Dietary Supplements.
79. Schweigert BS, Sauberlich HE, Elvehjem CA, And Baumann CA. Dietary protein and the vitamin b6 content of mouse tissue. From the department of biochemistry, college of agriculture, university of Wisconsin, Madison. May 20, 1946.
80. Abosamak NER, Gupta V. Vitamin B6 (Pyridoxine) [Updated 2023 Aug 17]. In: StatPearls [Internet]. Treasure Island (FL): StatPearls Publishing; 2023 Aug 17.
81. Brown MJ, Ameer MA, Daley SF, et al. Vitamin B6 Deficiency. [Updated 2023 Aug 8]. In: StatPearls [Internet]. Treasure Island (FL): StatPearls Publishing; 2023 Aug 8.
82. Getting Heme into Hemoglobin. NIH: National Institute of Diabetes and Digestive and Kidney Diseases. Aug 26, 2014.
83. Li C, Huang J, Zhu H, Shi Q, Li D, Ju X. Pyridoxal-5'-Phosphate Promotes Immunomodulatory Function of Adipose-Derived Mesenchymal Stem Cells through Indoleamine 2,3-Dioxygenase-1 and TLR4/NF-κB Pathway. Stem Cells Int. 2019 Nov 25;2019:3121246. doi: 10.1155/2019/3121246. PMID: 31885603; PMCID: PMC6899265.
84. Pyridoxine. Linus Pauling Institute. Micronutrient Information Center.
85. Harvey JW. Hematopoiesis. Veterinary Hematology, 2012.
86. Selhub J. Homocysteine metabolism. Annu Rev Nutr. 1999;19:217-46. doi: 10.1146/annurev.nutr.19.1.217. PMID: 10448523.
87. Hsu CC, Cheng CH, Hsu CL, Lee WJ, Huang SC, Huang YC. Role of vitamin B6 status on antioxidant defenses, glutathione, and related enzyme activities in mice with homocysteine-induced oxidative stress. Food Nutr Res. 2015 Apr 29;59:25702. doi: 10.3402/fnr.v59.25702. PMID: 25933612; PMCID: PMC4417078.
88. Choi SW, Friso S. Vitamins B6 and cancer. Subcell Biochem. 2012;56:247-64. doi: 10.1007/978-94-007-2199-9_13. PMID: 22116703.
89. Wyatt KM, Dimmock PW, Jones PW, Shaughn O'Brien PM. Efficacy of vitamin B-6 in the treatment of premenstrual syndrome: systematic review. BMJ. 1999 May 22;318(7195):1375-81. doi: 10.1136/bmj.318.7195.1375. PMID: 10334745; PMCID: PMC27878.
90. Doll H, Brown S, Thurston A, Vessey M. Pyridoxine (vitamin B6) and the premenstrual syndrome: a randomized crossover trial. J R Coll Gen Pract. 1989 Sep;39(326):364-8. PMID: 2558186; PMCID: PMC1711872.
91. Food Data Central - US Department of Agriculture. Bulgur, Dry (Sr Legacy, 170688).

92. Vitamin B7 fact sheet for health professionals. National Institutes of Health – Office of Dietary Supplements.
93. Bistas KG, Tadi P. Biotin. [Updated 2023 Jul 3]. In: StatPearls [Internet]. Treasure Island (FL): StatPearls Publishing.
94. Dasgupta A. Biotin. Biotin and Other Interferences in Immunoassays. 2019
95. Lage R, López M. AMPK: a metabolic gauge regulating whole-body energy homeostasis. Trends in Molecular Medicine, 2008.
96. Tomlinson DJ, Mülling CH, Fakler TM. Formation of Keratins in the Bovine Claw: Roles of Hormones, Minerals, and Vitamins in Functional Claw Integrity, Journal of Dairy Science, Volume 87, Issue 4, 2004, Pages 797-809, ISSN 0022-0302.
97. Stanley JS, Griffin JB, Zempleni J. Biotinylation of histones in human cells Effects of cell proliferation. Eur. J. Biochem. 268, 5424–5429 (2001) q FEBS 2001
98. Walth CB, Wessman LL, Wipf A. Response to: "Rethinking biotin therapy for hair, nail, and skin disorders". Journal of the American Academy of Dermatology. Volume 79, Issue 6, E121-E124, December 2018.
99. Ichihara Y, Suga K, Fukui M, Yonetani N, Shono M, Nakagawa R, Kagami S. Serum biotin level during pregnancy is associated with fetal growth and preterm delivery. J Med Invest. 2020;67(1.2):170-173. doi: 10.2152/jmi.67.170. PMID: 32378602.
100. Greenway FL, Ingram DK, Ravussin E, Hausmann M, Smith SR, Cox L, Tomayko K, Treadwell BV. Loss of taste responds to high-dose biotin treatment. J Am Coll Nutr. 2011 Jun;30(3):178-81. doi: 10.1080/07315724.2011.10719958. PMID: 21896875; PMCID: PMC5666569.
101. Piraccini BM, Berardesca E, Fabbrocini G, Micali G, Tosti A. Biotin: overview of the treatment of diseases of cutaneous appendages and of hyperseborrhea. G Ital Dermatol Venereol. 2019 Oct;154(5):557-566. doi: 10.23736/S0392-0488.19.06434-4. PMID: 31638351.
102. Masaru M, Yoshio M, Yuji F. Therapeutic Evaluation of the Effect of Biotin on Hyperglycemia in Patients with Non-Insulin Dependent Diabetes Mellitus. Journal of Clinical Biochemistry and Nutrition, 1993, Volume 14, Issue 3, Pages 211-218, Released on J-STAGE Feb 25, 2010, Online ISSN 1880-5086, Print ISSN 0912-0009, https://doi.org/10.3164/jcbn.14.211.
103. Kennedy DO. B Vitamins and the Brain: Mechanisms, Dose and Efficacy--A Review. Nutrients. 2016 Jan 27;8(2):68. doi: 10.3390/nu8020068. PMID: 26828517; PMCID: PMC4772032.
104. Staggs CG, Sealey WM, McCabe BJ, Teague AM, Mock DM. Determination of the biotin content of select foods using accurate and sensitive HPLC/avidin binding. J Food Compost Anal. 2004 Dec;17(6):767-776. doi: 10.1016/j.jfca.2003.09.015. PMID: 16648879; PMCID: PMC1450323.

105. Watanabe T, Kioka M, Fukushima M, Morimoto M and Sawamura H. Biotin content table of select foods and biotin intake in Japanese. International Journal of Analytical Bio-Science Vol. 2, No 4 (2014).
106. Vitamins. Drug Center. Gujarat Technical University.
107. Folate Fact Sheet for Health Professionals. National Institutes of Health. Office of Dietary Supplements.
108. Mingruo G. Folic Acid, Vitamins and Minerals as Functional Ingredients. Functional Foods: Principles and Technology, 2009.
109. Folic acid and folate. Istituto Superiore di Sanità. EpiCentro - Epidemiology for public health. Mar 29 21.
110. Rezk B, Haenen G, Vijgh W, Bast A. Tetrahydrofolate and 5-methyltetrahydrofolate are folates with high antioxidant activity. Identification of the antioxidant pharmacophore,
111. FEBS Letters, Volume 555, Issue 3, 2003, Pages 601-605, ISSN 0014-5793. https://doi.org/10.1016/S0014-5793(03)01358-9.
112. Folic Acid Safety, Interactions, and Health Outcomes. CDC: Centers for Disease Control and Prevention. May 15, 2024.
113. Tjong E, Dimri M, Mohiuddin SS. Biochemistry, Tetrahydrofolate. [Updated 2023 Jun 26]. In: StatPearls [Internet]. Treasure Island (FL): StatPearls Publishing;
114. Johnson L, Folate Deficiency (Folic Acid), University of Arkansas for Medical Sciences Reviewed/Revised Nov 2022. MSD Manual Professional version.
115. Lambie DG, Johnson RH. Drugs and folate metabolism. Drugs. 1985 Aug;30(2):145-55. doi: 10.2165/00003495-198530020-00003. PMID: 3896745.
116. Sahar, Saniya. (2021). Role of Folate and Folic Acid During Pregnancy. International Journal for Research in Applied Science and Engineering Technology. 9. 1488-1492. 10.22214/ijraset.2021.39295.
117. Borradale D, Isenring E, Hacker E, Kimlin MG. Exposure to solar ultraviolet radiation is associated with a decreased folate status in women of childbearing age. Journal of Photochemistry and Photobiology B: Biology, Volume 131, 2014, Pages 90-95, ISSN 1011-1344. https://doi.org/10.1016/j.jphotobiol.2014.01.002.
118. Knowles L, Morris AA, Walter JH. Treatment with Mefolinate (5-Methyltetrahydrofolate), but Not Folic Acid or Folinic Acid, Leads to Measurable 5-Methyltetrahydrofolate in Cerebrospinal Fluid in Methylenetetrahydrofolate Reductase Deficiency. JIMD Rep. 2016;29:103-107. doi: 10.1007/8904_2016_529. Epub 2016 Feb 23. Erratum in: JIMD Rep. 2016;29:117. doi: 10.1007/8904_2016_574. PMID: 26898294; PMCID: PMC5059208.

119. Liew SC, Gupta E. Methylenetetrahydrofolate reductase (MTHFR) C677T polymorphism: Epidemiology, metabolism and the associated diseases. European Journal of Medical Genetics, 2015.
120. Świgło A. Folates as antioxidants, Food Chemistry, Volume 101, Issue 4, 2007. Pages 1480-1483. ISSN 0308-8146. https://doi.org/10.1016/j.foodchem.2006.04.022.
121. Asbaghi O, Ghanavati M, Ashtary-Larky D, Bagheri R, Rezaei Kelishadi M, Nazarian B, Nordvall M, Wong A, Dutheil F, Suzuki K, et al. Effects of Folic Acid Supplementation on Oxidative Stress Markers: A Systematic Review and Meta-Analysis of Randomized Controlled Trials. Antioxidants. 2021; 10(6):871. https://doi.org/10.3390/antiox10060871
122. Asbaghi O, Ashtary-Larky D, Bagheri R, Moosavian SP, Nazarian B, Afrisham R, Kelishadi MR, Wong A, Dutheil F, Suzuki K, Alavi Naeini A. Effects of Folic Acid Supplementation on Inflammatory Markers: A Grade-Assessed Systematic Review and Dose-Response Meta-Analysis of Randomized Controlled Trials. Nutrients. 2021 Jul 6;13(7):2327. doi: 10.3390/nu13072327. PMID: 34371837; PMCID: PMC8308638.
123. Rashid S, Fareed M. Mechanistic view of folic acid on oral ulcers and oral cancers. Oral Oncology Reports. Volume 10, 2024, 100327, ISSN 2772-9060. https://doi.org/10.1016/j.oor.2024.100327.
124. Cueto HT, Riis AH, Hatch EE, Wise LA, Rothman KJ, Sørensen HT, Mikkelsen EM. Folic acid supplement use and menstrual cycle characteristics: a cross-sectional study of Danish pregnancy planners. Ann Epidemiol. 2015 Oct;25(10):723-9.e1. doi: 10.1016/j.annepidem.2015.05.008. Epub 2015 Jun 4. PMID: 26123570; PMCID: PMC4567938.
125. Miller AL. The methylation, neurotransmitter, and antioxidant connections between folate and depression. Altern Med Rev. 2008 Sep;13(3):216-26. PMID: 18950248.
126. Fooddata central. US department of agriculture. Avocados, raw.
127. Vitamin B12 Fact Sheet for Health Professionals. National Institutes of Health. Office of Dietary Supplements.
128. KS, Amarasena S, Mayengbam S. B Vitamins and Their Roles in Gut Health. Microorganisms. 2022 Jun 7;10(6):1168. doi: 10.3390/microorganisms10061168. PMID: 35744686; PMCID: PMC9227236.
129. Kundra P, Geirnaert A, Pugin B, Morales Martinez P, Lacroix C, Greppi A. Healthy adult gut microbiota sustains its own vitamin B12 requirement in an in vitro batch fermentation model. Front Nutr. 2022 Dec 1;9:1070155. doi: 10.3389/fnut.2022.1070155. PMID: 36532531; PMCID: PMC9751363.
130. Gupta ES, Sheth SP, Ganjiwale JD. Association of Vitamin B12 Deficiency and Use of Reverse Osmosis Processed Water for

Drinking: A Cross-Sectional Study from Western India. J Clin Diagn Res. 2016 May;10(5):OC37-40. doi: 10.7860/JCDR/2016/19621.7864. Epub 2016 May 1. PMID: 27437269; PMCID: PMC4948445.

131. Total dissolved solids in drinking water Background document for development of WHO Guidelines for Drinking-water Quality. WHO/SDE/WSH/03.04/16

132. Osman D, Cooke A, Young TR, Deery E, Robinson NJ, Warren MJ. The requirement for cobalt in vitamin B12: A paradigm for protein metalation. Biochim Biophys Acta Mol Cell Res. 2021 Jan;1868(1):118896. doi: 10.1016/j.bbamcr.2020.118896. Epub 2020 Oct 21. PMID: 33096143; PMCID: PMC7689651.

133. Johnson L. Vitamin B12 Deficiency (Pernicious Anemia). University of Arkansas for Medical Sciences. MSD Manual Professional Version. Nov 2022.

134. Vitamin B12–Deficiency Anemia. NIH- National Heart, Lung, and Blood Institute.

135. Barbosa L, Leal I, Timóteo AT, Matias T. Anemia megaloblástica aguda por inalação de óxido nitroso em doente com patologia autoimune múltipla [Acute megaloblastic anemia caused by inhalation of nitrous oxide in a patient with multiple autoimmune pathology]. Acta Med Port. 2000 Sep-Dec;13(5-6):309-12. Portuguese. PMID: 11234497.

136. Banihani SA. Vitamin B12 and Semen Quality. Biomolecules. 2017 Jun 9;7(2):42. doi: 10.3390/biom7020042. PMID: 28598359; PMCID: PMC5485731.

137. Sangle P, Sandhu O, Aftab Z, Anthony AT, Khan S. Vitamin B12 Supplementation: Preventing Onset and Improving Prognosis of Depression. Cureus. 2020 Oct 26;12(10):e11169. doi: 10.7759/cureus.11169. PMID: 33251075; PMCID: PMC7688056.

138. Agrawala, Ritesh Kumar; Sahoo, Srikanta Kumar; Choudhury, Arun Kumar; Mohanty, Binoy Kumar; Baliarsinha, Anoj Kumar. Pigmentation in vitamin B12 deficiency masquerading Addison's pigmentation: A rare presentation. Indian Journal of Endocrinology and Metabolism 17(Suppl1):p S254-S256, October 2013. | DOI: 10.4103/2230-8210.119591.

139. Raymond R. RussellIII, Heinrich Taegtmeyer. Anaplerosis- Encyclopedia of Biological Chemistry, 2004.

140. Halczuk K, Kaźmierczak-Barańska J, Karwowski BT, Karmańska A, Cieślak M. Vitamin B12-Multifaceted In Vivo Functions and In Vitro Applications. Nutrients. 2023 Jun 13;15(12):2734. doi: 10.3390/nu15122734. PMID: 37375638; PMCID: PMC10305463.

141. Halczuk K, Kaźmierczak-Barańska J, Karwowski BT, Karmańska A, Cieślak M. Vitamin B12—Multifaceted In Vivo Functions and In Vitro Applications. Nutrients. 2023; 15(12):2734. https://doi.org/10.3390/nu15122734

142. Domínguez-López I, Kovatcheva M, Casas R, Toledo E, Fitó M, Ros E, Estruch R, Serrano M, Lamuela-Raventós RM. Higher circulating vitamin B12 is associated with lower levels of inflammatory markers in individuals at high cardiovascular risk and in naturally aged mice. J Sci Food Agric. 2024 Jan 30;104(2):875-882. doi: 10.1002/jsfa.12976. Epub 2023 Sep 19. PMID: 37690097.

143. Altun, Idiris M; Kurutaş, Ergül Belge2. Vitamin B complex and vitamin B12 levels after peripheral nerve injury. Neural Regeneration Research 11(5):p 842-845, May 2016. | DOI: 10.4103/1673-5374.177150.

144. Brescoll J, Daveluy S. A review of vitamin B12 in dermatology. Am J Clin Dermatol. 2015 Feb;16(1):27-33. doi: 10.1007/s40257-014-0107-3. PMID: 25559140.

145. Valizadeh M, Valizadeh N. Obsessive compulsive disorder as early manifestation of B12 deficiency. Indian J Psychol Med. 2011 Jul;33(2):203-4. doi: 10.4103/0253-7176.92051. PMID: 22345852; PMCID: PMC3271502.

146. Collins EB, Yaguchi M. Vitamin B12 In Wheys Prepared by Coagulating Milk with Acid and Rennet. Department of Food Science and Technology, University of California, Davis.

147. Bito T, Okumura E, Fujishima M, Watanabe F. Potential of Chlorella as a Dietary Supplement to Promote Human Health. Nutrients. 2020 Aug 20;12(9):2524. doi: 10.3390/nu12092524. PMID: 32825362; PMCID: PMC7551956.

148. Genchi G, Lauria G, Catalano A, Carocci A, Sinicropi MS. Prevalence of Cobalt in the Environment and Its Role in Biological Processes. Biology (Basel). 2023 Oct 16;12(10):1335. doi: 10.3390/biology12101335. PMID: 37887045; PMCID: PMC10604320.

149. Vlasova AN, Kandasamy S, Chattha KS, Rajashekara G, Saif LJ. Comparison of probiotic lactobacilli and bifidobacteria effects, immune responses and rotavirus vaccines and infection in different host species. Vet Immunol Immunopathol. 2016 Apr;172:72-84. doi: 10.1016/j.vetimm.2016.01.003. Epub 2016 Jan 14. PMID: 26809484; PMCID: PMC4818210.

150. Reissig GN, Oliveira TFC. Fermented vegetables and fruits as vitamin B12 sources. International Food Research Journal 30(5): 1093 - 1104 (October 2023).

151. González-Montaña JR, Escalera-Valente F, Alonso AJ, Lomillos JM, Robles R, Alonso ME. Relationship between Vitamin B12 and Cobalt Metabolism in Domestic Ruminant: An Update. Animals (Basel). 2020 Oct 12;10(10):1855. doi: 10.3390/ani10101855. PMID: 33053716; PMCID: PMC7601760.

152. Bito T, Okumura E, Fujishima M, Watanabe F. Potential of Chlorella as a Dietary Supplement to Promote Human Health.

Nutrients. 2020 Aug 20;12(9):2524. doi: 10.3390/nu12092524. PMID: 32825362; PMCID: PMC7551956.

153. Payal, Lonkar & Payel, Karmakar & Walhe, Rajan. (2021). Traditionally Fermented Foods as Source of Vitamin B12 Producing LAB. LS International Journal of Life Sciences. 9. 162-168.

154. Christian AM, Krishnaveni GV, Kehoe SH, Veena SR, Khanum R, Marley-Zagar E, Edwards P, Margetts BM, Fall CH. Contribution of food sources to the vitamin B12 status of South Indian children from a birth cohort recruited in the city of Mysore. Public Health Nutr. 2015 Mar;18(4):596-609. doi: 10.1017/S1368980014000974. Epub 2014 May 27. PMID: 24866058; PMCID: PMC4266598.

155. Vitamin C Fact Sheet for Health Professionals. National Institutes of Health -Office of Dietary Supplements.

156. Ong J, Randhawa R. Scurvy in an alcoholic patient treated with intravenous vitamins. BMJ Case Rep. 2014 Apr 11;2014:bcr2013009479. doi: 10.1136/bcr-2013-009479. PMID: 24728889; PMCID: PMC3987238.

157. Márquez M, Rincón M, Sútil R, de Yépez CR, Saer R, Ponte S. Niveles séricos de vitamina C en adultos jóvenes consumidores crónicos de drogas de abuso [Serum levels of vitamin C in young adults who chronically use drugs of abuse]. Invest Clin. 2001 Sep;42(3):183-94. Spanish. PMID: 11552507.

158. Larry J. Vitamin C Deficiency (Scurvy). MSD Manual Professional Version.

159. Tembunde Y, Ge S, Turney K, Driscoll M. Scurvy: A Diagnosis Not to Be Missed. Cureus. 2022 Dec 28;14(12):e33050. doi: 10.7759/cureus.33050. PMID: 36721542; PMCID: PMC9881687.

160. Mayland CR, Bennett MI, Allan K. Vitamin C deficiency in cancer patients. Palliat Med. 2005 Jan;19(1):17-20. doi: 10.1191/0269216305pm970oa. PMID: 15690864.

161. Padayatty SJ, Katz A, Wang Y, Eck P, Kwon O, Lee JH, Chen S, Corpe C, Dutta A, Dutta SK, Levine M. Vitamin C as an antioxidant: evaluation of its role in disease prevention. J Am Coll Nutr. 2003 Feb;22(1):18-35. doi: 10.1080/07315724.2003.10719272. PMID: 12569111.

162. Paolini M, Pozzetti L, Pedulli GF, Marchesi E, Cantelli-Forti G. The nature of prooxidant activity of vitamin C. Life Sci. 1999;64(23):PL 273-8. doi: 10.1016/s0024-3205(99)00167-8. PMID: 10372660.

163. Boyera N, Galey I, Bernard BA. Effect of vitamin C and its derivatives on collagen synthesis and cross-linking by normal human fibroblasts. Int J Cosmet Sci. 1998 Jun;20(3):151-8. doi: 10.1046/j.1467-2494.1998.171747.x. PMID: 18505499.

164. DePhillipo NN, Aman ZS, Kennedy MI, Begley JP, Moatshe G, LaPrade RF. Efficacy of Vitamin C Supplementation on Collagen

Synthesis and Oxidative Stress After Musculoskeletal Injuries: A Systematic Review. Orthop J Sports Med. 2018 Oct 25;6(10):2325967118804544.

165. Pullar JM, Carr AC, Vissers MCM. The Roles of Vitamin C in Skin Health. Nutrients. 2017 Aug 12;9(8):866. doi: 10.3390/nu9080866. PMID: 28805671; PMCID: PMC5579659.

166. Carr AC, Maggini S. Vitamin C and Immune Function. Nutrients. 2017 Nov 3;9(11):1211. doi: 10.3390/nu9111211. PMID: 29099763; PMCID: PMC5707683.

167. Moores J. Vitamin C: a wound healing perspective. Br J Community Nurs. 2013 Dec;Suppl:S6, S8-11. doi: 10.12968/bjcn.2013.18.sup12.s6. PMID: 24796079.

168. Lynch SR, Cook JD. Interaction of vitamin C and iron. Ann N Y Acad Sci. 1980;355:32-44. doi: 10.1111/j.1749-6632.1980.tb21325.x. PMID: 6940487.

169. Hegsted DM, Finch CA, Kinney TD. The influence of diet on iron absorption; the interrelation of iron and phosphorus. J Exp Med. 1949 Aug 1;90(2):147-56. doi: 10.1084/jem.90.2.147. PMID: 18136194; PMCID: PMC2135900.

170. Peters, T., Apt, L., & Ross, J. F. (1971). Effect of Phosphates Upon Iron Absorption Studied in Normal Human Subjects and in Experimental Model Using Dialysis. Gastroenterology, 61(3), 315-322. https://doi.org/10.1016/S0016-5085(19)33527-9.

171. Sim M, Hong S, Jung S, Kim JS, Goo YT, Chun WY. Vitamin C supplementation promotes mental vitality in healthy young adults: results from a cross-sectional analysis and a randomized, double-blind, placebo-controlled trial. Eur J Nutr. 2022 Feb;61(1):447-459. doi: 10.1007/s00394-021-02656-3. Epub 2021 Sep 2.

172. Zylinska L, Lisek M, Guo F, Boczek T. Vitamin C Modes of Action in Calcium Involved Signaling in the Brain. Antioxidants. 2023; 12(2):231. https://doi.org/10.3390/antiox12020231.

173. Takeda N, Morita M, Hasegawa S, Horii A, Kubo T, Matsunaga T. Neuropharmacology of motion sickness and emesis. A review. Acta Otolaryngol Suppl. 1993;501:10-5.

174. Jarisch R, Weyer D, Ehlert E, Koch CH, Pinkowski E, Jung P, Kähler W, Girgensohn R, Kowalski J, Weisser B, Koch A. Impact of oral vitamin C on histamine levels and seasickness. J Vestib Res. 2014;24(4):281

175. Acerola (West Indian Cherry), Raw (Sr Legacy, 171686). Food Data Central. US Department of Agriculture Agricultural Research Service.

176. Assis, Sandra & Fernandes, Pedro & Martins, Antonio & Oliveira, Olga. (2008). Acerola: Importance, culture conditions, production and biochemical aspects.

177. Goraya RK, Bajwa U. Enhancing the functional properties and nutritional quality of ice cream with processed amla (Indian gooseberry). J Food Sci Technol. 2015 Dec;52(12):7861-71.

178. Peppers, Bell, Red, Raw (Foundation, 2258590). Food Data Central. US Department of Agriculture Agricultural Research Service.

179. Peppers, Bell, Yellow, Raw (Foundation, 2258589). Food Data Central. US Department of Agriculture Agricultural Research Service.

180. Peppers, Bell, Green, Raw (Foundation, 2258588). Food Data Central. US Department of Agriculture Agricultural Research Service.

181. Kiwifruit, Green, Raw (Sr Legacy, 168153). Food Data Central. US Department of Agriculture Agricultural Research Service.

182. Kiwifruit, Zespri Sungold, Raw (Sr Legacy, 168211. Food Data Central. US Department of Agriculture Agricultural Research Service.

183. Rose Hips, wild (Northern Plains Indians. Food Data Central. US Department of Agriculture Agricultural Research Service.

184. Trych U, Buniowska M, Skąpska S, Starzonek S, Marszałek K. The Bioaccessibility of Antioxidants in Black Currant Puree after High Hydrostatic Pressure Treatment. Molecules. 2020 Aug 3;25(15):3544.

185. Oprica L, Bucsa C, Zamfirache MM. Ascorbic Acid Content of Rose Hip Fruit Depending on Altitude. Iran J Public Health. 2015 Jan;44(1):138-9. PMID: 26060787; PMCID: PMC4450003.

186. Masoumi SZ, Ataollahi M, Oshvandi K. Effect of Combined Use of Calcium and Vitamin B6 on Premenstrual Syndrome Symptoms: a Randomized Clinical Trial. J Caring Sci. 2016 Mar 1;5(1):67-73. doi: 10.15171/jcs.2016.007. PMID: 26989667; PMCID: PMC4794546.

187. Jacobs ST, Starkey P. Calcium carbonate and the premenstrual syndrome: Effects on premenstrual and menstrual symptoms. American Journal of Obstetrics and Gynecology. Volume 179, Issue 2, 1998, Pages 444-452, ISSN 0002-9378.

188. Golding, P.H. Experimental folate deficiency in human subjects: what is the influence of vitamin C status on time taken to develop megaloblastic anaemia? BMC Hematol 18, 13 (2018). https://doi.org/10.1186/s12878-018-0107-2.

189. Watson WS, Vallance BD, Muir MM, Hume R. The effect of megadose ascorbic acid ingestion on the absorption and retention of vitamin B12 in man. Scott Med J. 1982 Jul;27(3):240-3. doi: 10.1177/003693308202700309. PMID: 7112085.

190. Barfi or Burfi, Indian Dessert (Survey (Fndds), 2341103). Food Data Central US Department of Agriculture.

ABOUT THE AUTHOR

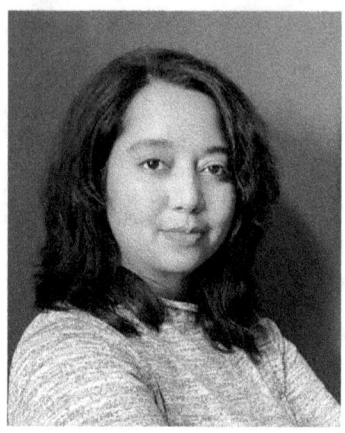

With a Master's Degree in Pharmacy, the author La Fonceur is a Research Scientist and Registered Pharmacist. She specialized in Pharmaceutical Technology and worked as a research scientist in the pharmaceutical research and development department. She is a health blogger and a dance artist. Her previous books include **Secret of Healthy Hair, Eat to Prevent and Control Disease,** and **Eat So What! series**. Being a research scientist, she has worked closely with drugs and based on her experience, she believes that one can prevent most of the diseases with nutritious vegetarian foods and a healthy lifestyle.

READ MORE FROM LA FONCEUR

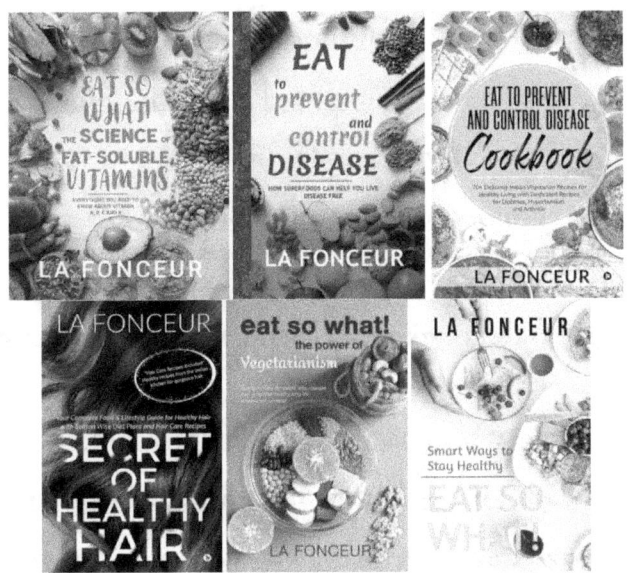

Hindi Editions

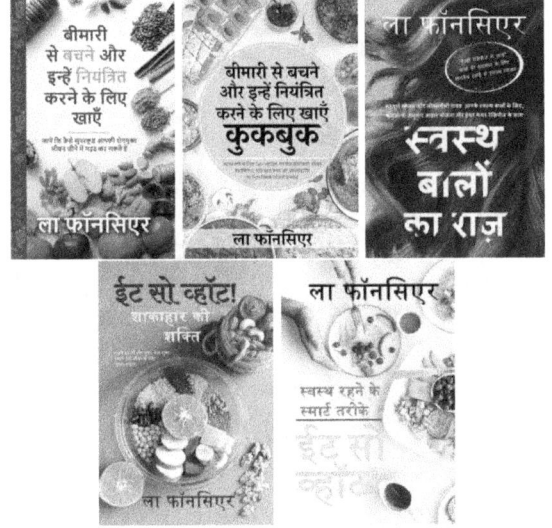

CONNECT WITH LA FONCEUR

Instagram: @la_fonceur | @eatsowhat

Facebook: LaFonceur | eatsowhatblog

Twitter: @la_fonceur

Follow on Bookbub: @eatsowhat

Sign up to get exclusive offers on La Fonceur books:

Blog: https://www.eatsowhat.com/

Website: https://www.lafonceurbooks.com/

Signed Copies: https://www.lafonceur.com/
(Ships to India only)

www.ingramcontent.com/pod-product-compliance
Lightning Source LLC
LaVergne TN
LVHW022233080526
838199LV00123B/621/J